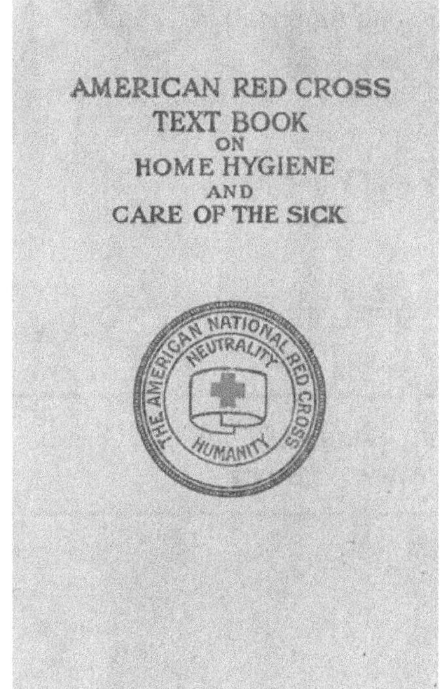

American Red Cross Text-Book on Home by Jane A. Delano and Anne Hervey Strong and American Red Cross

The Project Gutenberg EBook of American Red Cross Text-Book on Home

Title: American Red Cross Text-Book on Home Hygiene and Care of the Sick

AMERICAN RED CROSS TEXT-BOOK

ON

HOME CARE OF THE SICK

***

DELANO

AMERICAN RED CROSS

TEXT-BOOK

ON

HOME HYGIENE

AND

CARE OF THE SICK

BY

JANE A. DELANO, R. N.

Chairman of the National Committee, Red Cross Nursing Service; Director, Department of Nursing, American Red Cross; Late Superintendent of the Nurse Corps, U. S. A.; of the Training Schools for Nurses, Bellevue Hospital, New York City; and of the Training School for Nurses, Hospital of the University of Pennsylvania, Philadelphia

REVISED AND REWRITTEN

BY

ANNE HERVEY STRONG, R. N.

Professor of Public Health Nursing, Simmons College, Boston

This is the Second Edition of the American Red Cross Text-book in Elementary Hygiene and Home Care of the Sick by Jane A. Delano and Isabel McIsaac.

PREPARED FOR AND ENDORSED BY

THE AMERICAN RED CROSS

PHILADELPHIA P. BLAKISTON'S SON & CO.

1012 WALNUT STREET

COPYRIGHT, 1918, BY AMERICAN RED CROSS

THE MAPLE PRESS YORK PA

PREFACE

To the woman who wishes to protect her family from preventable diseases and is anxious to fit herself in the absence of a trained nurse to give intelligent care to those who are sick, this revision of the Red Cross text-book on Elementary Hygiene and Home Care of the Sick is particularly directed. It should appeal to men and to women who are interested in maintaining the health of their neighborhoods and communities and in affording effective coöperation to the public health authorities. To teachers wishing to impart protective health information to high school pupils, the book also should be useful as a class text as well as a guide.

The war, which has caused the withdrawal from private practice of thousands of physicians and graduate nurses, makes it peculiarly important to the nation for every adult to have sound knowledge as to how to prevent contagion and epidemics, especially by precautionary attention to home and local sanitation. With nurses becoming more difficult to secure, the safety of the family demands that some member in each household know enough about elementary nursing to make a patient comfortable and to carry out accurately the instructions of the physician.

The work of revision, based upon the latest knowledge of hygiene, sanitation and methods of home-nursing has been done by Miss Anne Hervey Strong, Professor of Public Health Nursing, Simmons College, under the personal direction of the author and the National Committee on Red Cross Nursing Service. The material has been painstakingly read by Dr. H. W. Rucker and Dr. Taliaferro Clarke of the United States Public Health Service, and Lieutenant Colonel Clarence H. Connor, Medical Corps, United States Army. Indebtedness to Dr. H. M. McCracken, President of Vassar College and Director of the Red Cross Junior Membership, for his valuable suggestion as to adapting the book for high school use as well as for the assistance rendered by his Department, also is gladly acknowledged.

J. A. D.

ACKNOWLEDGMENT

I wish to express my gratitude to those who have so kindly helped in the work of preparing the present edition. Thanks are especially due to Professor Isabel Stewart, Miss Anna C. Jamme, Professor Curtis M. Hilliard, Professor Maurice Bigelow, Miss Katharine Lord, Miss Josephine Goldmark, and Miss Evelyn Walker.

A. H. S.

CONTENTS

CHAPTER I

PAGE

CAUSES AND PREVENTION OF SICKNESS 1

Communicable diseases, 1. Micro-organisms and bacteria, 1. Parasites, 3. Structure and development of parasites, 4. Bacteria, 4. Shape, 4. Size, 5. Motion, 5. Multiplication, 5. Spores, 7. Distribution, 8. Protozoa, 8. Visible parasites, 8. Transmission of pathogenic organisms, 9. Defenses of the body, 12. Immunity, 13. Vaccination and inoculation, 15. Carriers, 17. Non-communicable diseases, 20. Physical examinations, 22.

CHAPTER II

HEALTH AND THE HOME 27

Heredity, 27. Hygiene of environment and person, 28. Ventilation, 29. Lighting, 32. Cleanliness of houses, 33. Garbage, 37. Insects, 38. Sewage, 39. Personal cleanliness, 41. Oral hygiene, 44. Treatment of teeth, 46. Clothing, 47. Food, 48. Elimination, 52. Rest and fatigue, 53. Sleep, 55. Recreation, 55.

CHAPTER III

BABIES AND THEIR CARE 60

Growth and development, 64. Average size, 64. Muscular development, 65. Development of special senses, of speech, of teeth, 66. Normal excretions, 67. Clothing, 68. Sleep, 70. Fresh air, 72. Diet, 72. Intervals of feeding, 73. Water, 75. Weaning, 75. Nursing bottles and nipples, 75. Tables of diet, 78. Bathing, 78. Eyes, 80. Mouth, 81. Nostrils, 81. Genital organs, 81. Development of habits, 82. Exercise, 83. Play and toys, 85.

CHAPTER IV

INDICATIONS OF SICKNESS 88

Objective symptoms, 92. Temperature, 92. Pulse, 96. Respiration, 99. General appearance, 100. Special senses, 101. Voice, tongue, throat, gums, 102. Cough, 103. Appetite, 103. Excretions, 103. Loss of weight, 104. Sleep, 104. Mental conditions, 104. Subjective symptoms, 105. Pain, 105. Records, 107. Tuberculosis, cancer and mental illness, 107. Tuberculosis, 109. Cancer, 111. Mental illness, 112.

CHAPTER V

EQUIPMENT AND CARE OF THE SICK ROOM 117

CHAPTER VI

BEDS AND BEDMAKING 132

CHAPTER VII

BATHS AND BATHING 154

Cleansing baths, 154. Bed bath, 156. Care of the mouth and teeth, 160. Care of the hair, 163. To wash the hair of a bed patient, 164. Hot foot-baths, 165. Cool sponge bath, 166.

CHAPTER VIII

APPLIANCES AND METHODS FOR THE SICK-ROOM 169

CHAPTER IX

FEEDING THE SICK 187

CHAPTER X

MEDICINES AND OTHER REMEDIES 200

CHAPTER XI

APPLICATION OF HEAT, COLD AND COUNTER-IRRITANTS 220

CHAPTER XII

CARE OF PATIENTS WITH COMMUNICABLE DISEASES 236

CHAPTER XIII

COMMON AILMENTS AND EMERGENCIES 257

CHAPTER XIV

SPECIAL POINTS IN THE CARE OF CHILDREN, CONVALESCENTS, CHRONICS, AND THE AGED 280

CHAPTER XV

INTRODUCTION

Health and sickness, at all times momentous factors in the welfare of our nation, now as never before are matters of vital importance. To win its victories both in peace and in war, the nation needs all its citizens with all their powers, and it is a matter of more than passing interest that, as conservative estimates show, at least three persons out of every hundred living in the United States are constantly incapacitated by serious sickness. In 1910 these seriously sick persons numbered more than 3,000,000. Even more significant, perhaps, is the fact that at least half of our national sickness could be prevented if knowledge and resources that we now possess were fully utilized.

The problem of sickness is by no means peculiar to our own day and generation. It has been a medical, a religious, and a social problem in every age. From the time of Job its meaning has baffled philosophers; from his day to ours thoughtful men have devoted their lives to searching for causes and cures. Yet before the middle of the last century little progress was made, either in scientific treatment or in prevention of disease.

The invention of the microscope first made possible a real understanding of sickness. Through the microscope a new world was revealed,--a world of the infinitely small, swarming with tiny forms of animal and vegetable life. No one, however, appreciated the significance of these hitherto invisible plants and animals until the latter part of the 19th century, when the great French savant, Pasteur, proved that little vegetable forms, now called bacteria, cause putrefaction and fermentation, and also certain diseases of animals and man. Pasteur's discoveries were carried still further by other scientists, with the result that bacteriology has revolutionized medicine, agriculture, and many industries, and has made possible the brilliant achievements of modern sanitary science. For the first time in history the prevention of epidemics has become possible, and sickness is no longer regarded as a punishment for sin.

Actual care of the sick, both in homes and in hospitals, has always been one of the responsibilities of women. The first general public hospital was built in Rome in the 4th century after Christ by Fabiola, a patrician lady. There she nursed the sick with her own hands, and from her day to ours extends an unbroken line of devoted women, handing down through the centuries their tradition of compassionate nursing service. It remained for Florence Nightingale, however, to give to the training its technical and scientific foundation, and thus to found the profession of nursing. As a result of her work, effectiveness was added to the spirit of service, that spirit which inspires the modern nurse no less than in an earlier day it inspired the Sisters of Charity who died nursing the wounded on the battlefields of Poland.

But different generations have different needs, and to meet them the spirit of service must manifest itself in widely varying ways. The sick need care today no less than they did when St. Elizabeth bathed the feet of the lepers; but such limited service, however beautiful, is no longer enough. Today we serve best by preventing sickness. Cure of sickness and alleviation of suffering must never be neglected; not in cure, however, but in prevention lies the hope of modern sanitary science, of modern medicine, and of modern nursing.

Nearly every woman at some time in her life is called upon to assist in caring for the sick. Indeed, approximately 90% of all sick persons in the United States are cared for at home, even in cities where hospital facilities are good. Moreover, every woman is largely responsible for maintaining her own health, and few escape responsibility at some time for maintaining the health of others. For such responsibility most women are poorly prepared. Every year in our own country thousands of persons, many of them babies and children, die merely because someone, in many cases a woman, is fatally ignorant of the laws governing sickness and health.

Only prolonged and careful training, such as good hospital training-schools afford, can furnish the skill and judgment required in nursing persons who are seriously ill. Upon the trained nurse the modern practice of medicine makes great and ever-increasing demands: a nurse must perform complicated duties, meet critical situations, and carry out a wide variety of measures based on scientific principles which she must understand. Good will and sympathy are no longer enough; amateur nursing, even when performed with the best intentions, may involve grave dangers for those who are seriously ill.

On the other hand, although it is true that a little knowledge is a dangerous thing, it is no less true that total ignorance may be more dangerous still. For instance, in cases of incipient, slight, or chronic illness, and in certain emergencies a little knowledge may be safer far than no knowledge at all; and no one, surely, should be ignorant of the principles of hygiene.

The American Red Cross, recognizing the part that women can and should play in preventing sickness and in building up the health and vigor of the nation, has added to its larger patriotic services this elementary course of instruction in hygiene and home care of the sick. The lessons are not intended to take the place of a nurse's training, and procedures requiring technical skill are necessarily omitted. The object of the book is to supply a little knowledge of sickness, which though limited may yet be safe. The book is also designed to set forth some general laws of health; to make possible earlier recognition of symptoms; to teach greater care in guarding against communicable disease; and to describe some elementary methods of caring for the sick, which, however simple, are essential to comfort, and sometimes indeed to ultimate recovery.

FOR FURTHER READING

A History of Nursing--Dock and Nutting, Volume I.

The Life of Florence Nightingale--Cook.

The Life of Pasteur--Vallery-Radot.

The House on Henry Street--Wald.

Public Health Nursing--Gardner, Part I, Chapters I-III.

Origin and Growth of the Healing Art--Berdoe.

Medical History from the Earliest Times--Withington.

Under the Red Cross Flag--Boardman.

Report on National Vitality--Fisher, (Bulletin 30 of the Committee of One Hundred on National Health. Government Printing Office, Washington).

CHAPTER I

CAUSES AND PREVENTION OF SICKNESS

Diseases of two kinds have long been recognized: first, those transmitted directly or indirectly from person to person, like smallpox, measles, and typhoid fever; and second, diseases like heart disease and apoplexy, which are not so transmitted. These two classes are popularly called "catching" and "not catching;" the former are the infectious or communicable diseases, and the latter the non-infectious or non-communicable. The term contagious, formerly applied to diseases supposed to be spread only by direct contact, is no longer an accurate or useful term.

THE COMMUNICABLE DISEASES

The invention of the microscope, as we have seen, revealed the existence of innumerable little plants and animals, so small that even many millions crowded together are invisible to the naked eye. These tiny living creatures are called micro-organisms or germs. The plant forms are called bacteria (singular, bacterium), and the animal forms protozoa (singular, protozoön). The common belief that all or even most bacteria are harmful is quite unfounded. As a matter of fact, while not less than 1500 different kinds of micro-organisms or germs are known, only about 75 varieties are known to produce disease.

Most bacteria belong to the class of micro-organisms called saprophytes, which find their food in dead organic matter, both animal and vegetable, and cannot flourish in living tissues. These saprophytes act upon the tissues of dead animals and vegetables, and resolve them into simpler substances, which are then ready to serve as nourishment for plants higher in the vegetable kingdom. Thus the processes which we know as fermentation and putrefaction are due to the action of saprophytes. Higher plants in turn furnish food for men and animals, and so the food supply is used over and over in different forms, making what is known as the *food cycle*. If it were not for bacterial activities vegetation would be robbed of its supply of nourishment, and plant life would speedily end; destruction of plant life would deprive the animal kingdom of food and thus all life would become extinct. The saprophytes are consequently essential to the existence of both animals and vegetables.

There are, however, other organisms called *parasites*, which can exist in living tissues of animals or vegetables. The organisms at whose expense the parasites live are called their *hosts*. Parasites not only contribute nothing to their hosts, but generally harm them by producing poisonous substances or depriving them of food. Some parasites are able to lead a saprophytic existence also, but as a rule they live at the expense of animal or plant life. Pathogenic, or disease-producing, germs belong to the group of parasites. The pathogenic germs which find favorable soil in the body produce poisons called toxins. These poisons or toxins interfere with the bodily functions, and thus cause what we know as communicable disease. Communicable diseases are caused by specific germs only: that is, a certain disease cannot develop unless its particular germs are present; the germs of typhoid for instance, can cause typhoid fever only, and not tuberculosis or other disease.

A number of diseases are caused by micro-organisms that are now well known. Chief among these diseases are colds, septicæmia (blood poisoning), influenza, pneumonia, diphtheria, typhoid fever, tuberculosis, whooping cough, Asiatic cholera, bubonic plague, meningitis, tetanus ("lock jaw"), leprosy, gonorrhoea, syphilis, relapsing fever, typhus fever, glanders, and anthrax. Micro-organisms not yet identified probably cause the communicable diseases whose origin is not known with certainty. These include infantile paralysis, smallpox, scarlet fever, measles, mumps, chicken-pox, Rocky Mountain spotted fever, yellow fever, hydrophobia (rabies), foot-and-mouth disease. We can hardly doubt that the intensive laboratory research now in progress will reveal in the near future the specific germs of these diseases also.

STRUCTURE AND DEVELOPMENT OF PARASITES

The group of parasites consists of two general classes, the vegetable, and the animal. In the former class belong the bacteria, and in the latter the protozoa. The two classes are not sharply differentiated, but in general the vegetable parasites are less highly organized than the animal.

BACTERIA

SHAPE.--Bacteria are composed of single cells and are consequently called unicellular organisms. Under the microscope individual cells are seen to differ in size, shape, and structure. In shape bacteria show three different types; the rod-shaped (bacillus), the spherical (coccus), and the spiral (spirillum). The organisms causing typhoid fever for example are a variety of bacilli, those causing pneumonia are cocci, while those causing Asiatic cholera are spirilla.

[Illustration: FIG. 1.--BACILLI OF VARIOUS FORMS. (*Williams.*)]

SIZE.--Bacteria vary greatly in size. Average rod-shaped bacteria are about 1/25000 of an inch long, but there are undoubtedly organisms so small that they cannot be seen, even by means of the strongest microscopes we now possess.

[Illustration: STAPHYLOCOCCI. STREPTOCOCCI. DIPLOCOCCI. TETRADS. SARCINÆ. FIG. 2.--(*Williams.*)]

MOTION.--The power of motion in certain species of bacteria is due to hair-like appendages called flagella. These flagella by a lashing movement somewhat resembling the action of oars enable the organisms to move through fluids.

MULTIPLICATION.--After bacteria have fully developed, each cell divides into two equal parts; the process of division is called fission. Each of these two parts rapidly grows into a full-sized organism. Then fission again takes place, so that four bacteria replace the original one. In each of the four, fission occurs again, and so the process of multiplication continues. As bacteria develop they group themselves in characteristic ways. Some, like the streptococci, arrange themselves in chains; the diplococci, in pairs; the tetrads, in groups of four; others in packets called sarcinæ, and still others, the staphylococci, form masses supposed to resemble bunches of grapes.

[Illustration: FIG. 3.--SPIRILLA OF VARIOUS FORMS. (*Williams.*)]

[Illustration: FIG. 4.--BACTERIA SHOWING FLAGELLA. (*Williams.*)]

Under favorable conditions fission occurs rapidly; in some types a new generation may appear as often as every 15 minutes. Enormous multiplication would result if nothing occurred to check the process. But in nature such increase never continues unhindered, and bacteria, acting upon their food substances, produce acids and other materials injurious to themselves. Furthermore, lack of proper food, moisture, or favorable temperature, and competition with other organisms tend to prevent their unrestricted growth and multiplication.

[Illustration: FIG. 5.--BACTERIA WITH SPORES. (*Williams.*)]

SPORES.--Most bacteria die if conditions become unfavorable to their growth, but some enter into a resting stage. This stage is characterized by the development of round or oval glistening bodies called spores, which are of dense structure and possess an extraordinary power to withstand heat, chemicals, and unfavorable surroundings. Except in rare instances a single cell produces but one spore. As soon as favorable conditions of temperature, moisture, and food supply are restored, the spore develops into the active form of the germ; it may, however, remain dormant for months or years. Spore formation, however, occurs in only a very few varieties of pathogenic bacteria.

DISTRIBUTION.--Bacteria are very widely distributed in nature; they are in fact found practically everywhere on the surface of the earth. They are present in plants and water and food; on fabrics and furniture, walls and floors; and they are found in great numbers on the skin, hair, many mucous surfaces, and other tissues of the body.

PROTOZOA

The protozoa are the lowest group of the animal kingdom. Like bacteria they are composed of single cells so small as to be visible only under the microscope. They play an important part in causing certain diseases of man, especially in the tropics. Among the well-known human diseases of protozoan origin are malaria, amoebic dysentery, and sleeping-sickness. Protozoa also cause several wide-spread and serious plagues of domestic animals.

VISIBLE PARASITES

A few diseases are caused by parasites large enough to be seen with the naked eye. One of the most important is hookworm disease. This disease is caused by a tiny worm which penetrates the victim's skin and ultimately finds its way into the intestine. Other diseases also are caused by parasitic worms, such as tapeworms, pinworms, and trichinæ. The latter are acquired as a result of eating infected meat, particularly infected pork that has not been thoroughly cooked.

TRANSMISSION OF PATHOGENIC ORGANISMS

Pathogenic or disease producing organisms need for their development food, moisture, darkness, and warmth, conditions that exist within the human body. When one or more of these factors is unfavorable, development of germs is checked; if unfavorable conditions are extreme or long continued, the organisms begin to die. It is difficult to say at exactly what moment they will die if deprived of moisture or exposed to extremes of temperature or other unfavorable conditions, just as it would be impossible to state at exactly what moment a collection of house plants would all be dead if water were withheld, or if the room temperature were greatly reduced.

Most pathogenic organisms, however, do not flourish long outside the body, and owe their continued existence to a fairly direct transfer from person to person. They gain access to the body through mucous surfaces such as the respiratory and digestive tracts, and through breaks in the skin, such as cuts, abrasions, and the bites of certain insects. They leave the body chiefly in the nasal and mouth discharges, as in coughing, sneezing, and spitting, in the urine and bowel discharges, and in pus or "matter."

[Illustration: FIG. 6. (*L. H. Wilder.*)]

The problem of controlling communicable diseases, consequently, lies in preventing the bodily discharges of one person from travelling directly into the body of another. If a person is not expelling pathogenic germs, it is clear that he cannot pass diseases on to others. But both pathogenic and harmless germs follow the same routes from person to person, so that safety as well as decency lies in preventing so far as possible all exchanges of bodily discharges.

There are five routes by which the bodily discharges most frequently travel from one person to another. Four of these routes of infection are called public, because in most cases efforts of individuals alone are not sufficient to control them. The public routes are water, milk, food, and insects. The fifth, or private route, includes all means by which fresh discharges of one person are passed to another, as when nose and mouth discharges are carried in coughing, sneezing, and kissing, or when bowel and bladder discharges are carried by the hands. These five routes in a given case differ greatly in relative importance, but the fifth, or direct route plays an immense part, although its importance in causing sickness has only lately been recognized. It cannot be too strongly emphasized that the chief agent in the spread of human diseases is man himself, and the human hand is the great carrier of disease germs both to and from the body. If unclean hands could be kept away from the orifices of the body, particularly the mouth, many diseases would soon cease to exist.

Defenses of the Body

In view of all the dangers from disease-producing germs it may seem surprising that the human race has not long ago succumbed to its invisible enemies. But the body has various defenses by means of which it may prevent invasion, or successfully combat its enemies in case they do gain access.

The unbroken skin is usually impassable to bacteria. Virulent organisms are often found upon the skin of perfectly healthy persons, where they appear to be harmless unless an abrasion occurs which affords entrance into the deeper tissues. Most bacteria breathed in with the air cling to the moist surfaces of the air-passages and never reach the lungs.

Mucous membranes lining the mouth and other cavities of the body would prove favorable sites for the growth of bacteria if the mucus secreted by them were not frequently removed. The mouth of a healthy person may contain bacteria of many kinds, but the saliva has a slight disinfectant power and serves as a constant wash to the membranes. The normal gastric (stomach) juice is decidedly unfavorable to the growth of bacteria, although it does not always kill them; they often pass through the stomach and are found in large numbers in the intestines. Other bodily secretions, such as the tears and perspiration, tend to discourage bacterial growth.

Tissues of the body vary greatly in their power to resist invading germs, so that the route by which germs enter influences the severity of their effects. Typhoid bacilli and the spirilla of Asiatic cholera when taken with food or water produce far more serious disturbances than when injected under the skin; infections from pus germs through an abrasion of the skin may result in a slight local disturbance, while the same amount introduced into a deeper wound might cause a fatal infection. Certain germs nourish in certain tissues only; even tuberculosis, which attacks practically all tissues, has its favorite locations.

IMMUNITY.--In addition to its mechanical defenses against disease, the body shows a varying degree of *immunity*, or the power possessed by living organisms to resist infections. Immunity or resistance is the opposite of susceptibility. It is exceedingly variable, being greater or less in different people and under different conditions, but the exact ways in which it is brought about are still in many cases far from clear.

Immunity may be *natural* or *acquired*. By natural immunity is meant an inherited characteristic by which all individuals of a species are immune to a certain disease. The natural immunity of certain species of animals to the diseases of other animals is well known. Man is immune to many diseases of lower animals, and they in turn are immune to many diseases of man. Cattle, for instance, are immune to typhoid and yellow fever, while man shows high resistance to rinderpest and Texas fever; both, however, are susceptible to tuberculosis, to which goats are immune. There are all gradations of immunity within the same species. Moreover, certain individuals have a personal immunity against diseases to which others of the same race or species are susceptible.

Immunity may be *acquired* in several ways. It is commonly known that one attack of certain communicable diseases renders the individual immune for a varying length of time, and sometimes for life. Among these diseases are smallpox, measles, whooping-cough, scarlet fever, infantile paralysis, typhoid fever, chicken-pox, and mumps; erysipelas and pneumonia on the other hand appear to diminish resistance and to leave a person more susceptible to later attacks.

Again, in some cases immunity may be artificially acquired by introducing certain substances into the body to increase its resistance. Examples of this method include the use of antitoxin as a protection against diphtheria, of sera in pneumonia and other infections, and vaccination against smallpox and typhoid fever whereby a slight form of the disease is artificially induced. Laboratory research goes on constantly, and doubtless many more substances will eventually be discovered that will reduce human misery as vaccines and antitoxin have already reduced it.

Vaccination and inoculation have saved thousands of lives. Smallpox, once more prevalent than measles, was the scourge of Europe until vaccination was introduced. During the 18th century it was estimated that 60,000,000 people died of it, and at the beginning of the 19th century one-fifth of all children born died of smallpox before they were 10 years old. In countries where vaccination is not practised the disease is as serious as ever; in Russia during the five years from 1893-97, 275,502 persons died of smallpox, while in Germany where vaccination is compulsory, only 8 people died of it during the year 1897. Death rates from diphtheria and typhoid fever have been greatly reduced by the use of antitoxin and antityphoid vaccine. Thus in New York State in 1894, before antitoxin was generally used, 99 out of every 100,000 of the population died of diphtheria, while only 20 out of 100,000 died of it in 1914. In 1911 a United States Army Division of more than 12,000 men camped at San Antonio, Texas, for four months. All of these men were vaccinated against typhoid fever and only a single case occurred during the summer, although conditions of camp life always tend to spread the disease.

While many and various factors tend to lower resistance rather than to increase it, the idea that these factors act equally in all kinds of infection is erroneous.

"The principal causes which diminish resistance to infection are: wet and cold, fatigue, insufficient or unsuitable food, vitiated atmosphere, insufficient sleep and rest, worry, and excesses of all kinds. The mechanism by which these varying conditions lower our immunity must receive our attention, for they are of the greatest importance in preventive medicine. It is a matter of common observation that exposure to wet and cold or sudden changes of temperature, overwork, worry, stale air, poor food, etc., make us more liable to contract certain diseases. The tuberculosis propaganda that has been spread broadcast with such energy and good effect has taught the value of fresh air and sunshine, good food, and rest in increasing our resistance to this infection.

"There is, however, a wrong impression abroad that because a lowering of the general vitality favors certain diseases, such as tuberculosis, common colds, pneumonia, septic and other infections, it plays a similar rôle in all communicable diseases. Many infections, such as smallpox, measles, yellow fever, tetanus, whooping-cough, typhoid fever, cholera, plague, scarlet fever, and other diseases, have no particular relation whatever to bodily vigor. These diseases often strike down the young and vigorous in the prime of life. The most robust will succumb quickly to tuberculosis if he receives a sufficient dose of the virulent micro-organisms. A good physical condition does not always temper the virulence of the disease; on the contrary, many infections run a particularly severe course in strong and healthy subjects, and, contrariwise, may be mild and benign in the feeble. Physical weakness, therefore, is not necessarily synonymous with increased susceptibility to all infections, although true for some of them. In other words, 'general debility' lowers resistance in a specific, rather than in a general, sense."--(Rosenau: Preventive Medicine and Hygiene, pp. 403 and 404.)

CARRIERS

Well persons who carry in their bodies pathogenic germs but who themselves have no symptoms of disease are called carriers. Thus typhoid carriers have typhoid bacilli in the intestinal tract, while they themselves show no symptoms of typhoid fever; diphtheria carriers have bacilli of diphtheria in the throat or nose, but have themselves no symptoms of diphtheria, and so on. It has now been proved that many patients harbor bacteria for weeks, months, or even years following an infection, and are dangerous distributors of disease; also, some healthy individuals without a history of illness harbor living bacteria which may infect susceptible persons in the usual ways. Transmission by healthy carriers goes far to explain the occurrence of diseases among persons who have apparently not been exposed. This explanation has greatly clarified the whole problem of the spread of communicable diseases. Carriers, unfortunately, exist in large numbers, and render the ultimate control of disease exceedingly difficult. They can usually be identified by bacteriological tests. To some extent they can be supervised; food handlers at least should be legally obliged to submit to physical examinations, and should be licensed only when proved free from communicable disease.

Diseases are also spread by persons suffering from them in a form so mild or so unusual that they pass unrecognized. These persons are known as "missed" cases. Carriers of disease and "missed" cases go freely about the community, handling food, using common drinking cups, travelling in crowded street cars, standing in crowded shops; in various ways coming into close contact with other people, coughing and sneezing and kissing their friends no less often than normal individuals. It is consequently clear that the bodily discharges of supposedly normal persons may be hardly less a menace than those of persons known to be infected.

Diseases that depend for transmission upon milk, water, food, and insects may be controlled by public action, that is, by specific measures taken by a large group of people in order to protect the individual. Such action constitutes *public sanitation*. There is, however, a large group of diseases, chiefly sputum-borne, that cannot be controlled except by individual action. Such individual action constitutes a large part of *personal hygiene*.

The whole problem of controlling infections sounds simple, depending as it does for the most part upon unpolluted water, milk, and food, extermination of certain insects, and cleanliness in personal behaviour.

In practice the problem is not so easy. Public sanitation has performed miracles in the past, and will do much in the future; behaviour, however, will continue to be influenced by many factors, social and economic as well as personal. Ignorance of the laws of health is an obstacle to progress, but in modern conditions even the instructed may be unable to control their ways of living and working. Indeed, such control is at present limited to the privileged few. On the ignorant and the poor, those least able to bear it, society loads the heaviest burden of sickness. Only when ignorance and poverty are abolished, as one day they will be, can the final stage be reached in the fight for public health.

THE NON-COMMUNICABLE DISEASES

In this group is included a great variety of maladies. Of some the causes are known, while in the case of others, origin, prevention, and remedy are still obscure. Here belong defects in structure of the body, both hereditary and acquired; insanity and other nervous diseases; new growths, like tumors and cancer; disturbances of bodily processes, as malnutrition and gout; and the important class of degenerative diseases, like arteriosclerosis, in which tissues become hardened and fibrous and hence less able to perform their normal functions.

The degenerative diseases are playing a menacing part in national health. The average length of life in the United States has shown a marked increase it is true, during the last 40 years. But this gain represents chiefly the saving of life through prevention of communicable diseases, especially among babies and children; among people who have passed the 30th year on the other hand, death rates are actually increasing. This increase is most marked after the age of 45, and is caused chiefly by the increase of cancer, and of degenerative diseases of the heart, blood vessels, and kidneys. Degeneration of tissues is normally a condition typical of old age, and in aged persons it may occur in any tissue. There is no elixir of youth, and for old age there is no cure. But the important facts in this connection are that degenerative changes now occur prematurely, and that among a vast number of people, in various classes of society and various occupations, the vital organs show a marked tendency to break down after the age of 45.

This condition is not inevitable. Before the beginning of the present war, death rates at all ages were decreasing in England, Sweden, and other European countries. In America also degenerative diseases can be checked or prevented to a large extent, and it is highly important that their causes should be generally understood.

The two groups following include some of the probable causes:

1. Conditions of life which result in continued overwork, and mental overwork in particular; worry, excitement, insufficient recreation and exercise, and other kinds of nervous strain typical of modern life, especially in cities.

2. Irritating substances in the body, including poisonous substances resulting from infectious diseases, and from syphilis in particular; poisons from chronic infections, alcohol, and industrial poisons such as lead and other metals; overeating and improper eating, especially of meat and other proteins, and rich or highly seasoned food; faulty digestion, constipation, and imperfect elimination through the kidneys.--(See Dr. A. E. Shipley, in bulletin of the N. Y. City Dept. of Health, Feb., 1915.)

The importance of early recognition cannot be overemphasized. In many of these troubles the symptoms are not pronounced, and the victims have no knowledge of their condition until they happen to be examined for life insurance, or until the disease is far advanced. And even when they realize that trouble exists, as for example constipation or overwork, most people absolutely fail to realize how serious the consequences may be. The first step toward remedy is periodic complete physical examination by a competent physician, in order to learn in time how to prevent these degenerative diseases, if present, from growing worse. The custom of undergoing an annual physical examination is becoming more common, and "such a course, conservatively estimated, would add 5 years to the average life of persons between 45 and 50."--(Winslow.)

"Recently, we have been making examinations of the employees of whole institutions, large banks and other industrial concerns in New York City, and we find almost the same conditions there. Out of 2000 such examinations among young men and women of an average age of 33, just in the early prime of life, men and women supposedly picked because of their especial fitness for work, only 3.14% were found free of impairment or of habits of living which are obviously leading to impairment. Of the remaining persons, 96.69% were unaware of impairment; 5.38% of the total number examined were affected with chronic heart trouble; 13.10% with arteriosclerosis; 25.81% with high or low blood pressure; 35.65% with sugar, casts or albumen in the urine; 12.77% with combination of both heart and kidney disease; 22.22% with decayed teeth or infected gums; 16.03% with faulty vision uncorrected.... The fact of greatest import, however, was that impairment, sufficiently serious to justify the examiner in referring the examinee to his family physician for medical treatment, was found in 59% of the total number of cases, while 37.86% were on the road to impairment because of the use of "too much alcohol," or "too much tobacco," constipation, eye-strain, overweight, diseased mouths, errors of diet, and so forth....

"And what is the cause of this appalling increase, in the United States, of these and other degenerative diseases? I believe it can be shown to the satisfaction of any reasonable person that the increase is largely due to the neglect of individual hygiene in United States....

"If a man were suddenly afflicted with smallpox or typhoid fever or any other acute malady, he would lose no time in getting expert advice and applying every known means to save his life. But his life may be threatened just as seriously, though possibly not so imminently, by arteriosclerosis, heart disease, or Bright's disease, and he will do nothing to prevent the encroachment of these diseases until it is too late, but will continue to eat as he pleases, drink as he pleases, smoke as he pleases, or overwork, and worry himself into a premature grave."--("Conservation of Life at Middle Age," Prof. Irving Fisher, Am. Journal of Public Health, July, 1915.)

Periodic physical examinations are as necessary for children as for adults, in order to detect physical defects. These defects are known to have such an immense bearing upon health that routine examinations of all children have become an integral part of the work of enlightened public schools.

Prevention of degenerative disease, then, as well as of the enormous numbers of preventable accidents and injuries, depends in large measure upon proper living conditions and proper personal habits. The infectious diseases, according to Dr. Hill, cost us annually at least 10 billion dollars in addition to the loss of life, and he adds: "The infectious diseases in general radiate from and are kept going by women."--(Hill--New Public Health, p. 30.) Women, it is true, can prevent many of the infections, but they can do still more, for hygienic habits to be effective must be acquired early, and mothers and teachers, because they have practically the entire control of children, have the power to prevent many cases of degenerative as well as of communicable disease.

EXERCISES

1. Distinguish between communicable and non-communicable disease.

2. Describe the part played by micro-organisms in causing disease.

3. Describe the structure of bacteria and their method of multiplication.

4. In what ways are pathogenic germs transmitted from person to person?

5. Upon what preventive measures does the control of communicable diseases depend?

6. What is meant by immunity?

7. Against what diseases may immunity be acquired artificially? How has the practice of immunizing affected death rates from communicable diseases?

8. What factors tend to lower resistance? Do they act equally in the case of all diseases?

9. Define a carrier, and explain the importance of carriers in the spread of disease.

10. Name some of the characteristics and causes of degenerative diseases.

11. Whom do the degenerative diseases most commonly affect?

12. Describe methods that should be employed to prevent degenerative diseases.

FOR FURTHER READING

The New Public Health--Hill, Chapters I-IX.

Health and Disease--Roger I. Lee, Chapters XV-XXIV.

Principles of Sanitary Science and the Public Health--Sedgwick, Chapters I, II, III.

Scientific Features of Modern Medicine--Frederic S. Lee, Chapters II, IV-VI.

Disease and Its Causes--Councilman, Chapter I.

Preventive Medicine and Hygiene--Rosenau.

Publications of the Life Extension Institute--25 West 45th Street, New York City.

CHAPTER II

HEALTH AND THE HOME

Of all the considerations that determine health, heredity is the one
unalterable factor. Although certain characteristics are obviously
hereditary,--complexion, height, and mental and physical traits in great
variety,--yet in the past heredity has been little understood. In
consequence it has served too often as a scape goat for faults and
failings not beyond an individual's control. Our first clear understanding
of the principles underlying heredity resulted from experiments made
by Mendel, an Austrian monk, during the last century, and it is now
possible to predict with a high degree of accuracy the inheritance of
certain characteristics.

Many diseases, formerly considered hereditary because their actual
causes were unknown, are now known to be communicable. Thus, it is
now understood that tuberculosis is not hereditary, although little
children may be infected by tuberculous parents. No germ diseases
are inherited in the strict sense of the word; but a baby may be infected
with syphilis before birth if his father or his mother has the disease.

It is true, however, that certain tissue weaknesses of the body seem to
be hereditary, and in consequence one family is more susceptible to
digestive disorders, another to diseases of the lungs, a third to
deafness, and so on. Moreover, general low vitality may be inherited. It
should be emphasized, however, that hereditary weakness does not
inevitably lead to disease. Many persons have succeeded in
preventing the development of active disease by guarding against
strain in directions where they are weak by inheritance.

Of all tissue weaknesses that may be inherited, defects of the nervous
system are the most serious. Nervous disorders of every degree of
severity, from slight nervous instability even to insanity, may result
when these tissues are defective; but it is now a recognized fact that
nervous disorders in many cases can be prevented from developing.
Feeblemindedness, another condition due to defective tissue, is known
to be inherited in the majority of cases, and in all cases it is incurable.

HYGIENE OF ENVIRONMENT AND PERSON

By environment is meant everything outside the body that affects it; taken in its complete meaning the word might include everything that is or ever was in the whole universe. It is possible to consider here a few only of the many environmental and personal factors affecting the health of individuals.

The home constitutes the important part of environment for most persons, and for children in particular, since they spend the greater part of their time in or about it, and get there the foundation on which their health in later years depends. For persons employed away from home, industrial and occupational hygiene is hardly less important; but those subjects are too extensive to be considered here.

Most people live where they must, and few have any part in planning the construction of their own houses. In choosing a house, however, one should remember that rooms where sunshine never enters are unfit for continued occupation. For children in particular fresh air and sunshine are essential, and it may be economy in the end to pay a comparatively high rent for an apartment having sunshine during at least a part of the day. Ignorance and carelessness, unfortunately, can spoil the best living conditions, and sometimes even in the country fresh air and sunshine are excluded from sleeping and living rooms.

VENTILATION.--Ventilation has a direct bearing on health, although, contrary to former belief, the actual amount of oxygen in the air is not ordinarily the most important factor; even badly ventilated rooms contain more than enough oxygen to support life. The factors of prime importance in ventilation are temperature, humidity, air movement, and the number of persons in a given space since the greater the distance from one another the less is the probability that diseases will be spread.

Room temperature should not be above 70° F. and, except for the aged or sick, it is better to be between 60° and 65°. Some moisture in the air is desirable; the amount needed is from 50% to 55% of the total moisture that the air can hold at a given temperature. We have no apparatus to decrease humidity in the air of houses, and in summer we are obliged to endure humidity, if excessive, no matter how uncomfortable we may be. But in winter the air in most houses is too dry, so that the mucous membranes of the nose and throat often become irritated and susceptible to infection. Most heating systems, particularly in small buildings, make no provision for supplying moisture. Keeping water in open dishes on or near radiators is often recommended, and would greatly improve the condition of the air, if people remembered to keep the dishes filled.

The following is a simple but effective device to increase humidity: Roll an ordinary desk blotter into a cone about 8 inches in diameter at the base, and keep it constantly submerged for about one inch in a dish of water. The water rises to the top of the blotter and a large surface for evaporation is thus afforded.

[Illustration: FIG. 7.]

Stagnant air is harmful. Air should be in constant though not necessarily perceptible motion. Air about the body, if motionless, acts like a warm moist blanket, preventing the passage of heat from the body.

The three factors, heating, humidity, and air motion, must be considered together. Every person requires each hour about 3000 cubic feet of air, and the problem of heating and ventilating is that of providing this amount in gentle motion, at a temperature of about 65° F., and of humidity from 50-55%. Higher temperatures and stagnant air cause disinclination to work, headache, nausea, restlessness, or sleepiness, and if continued are likely to result in loss of appetite, and anemia. The tuberculosis movement has clearly shown the benefits both for the sick and the well of living in the open air, and has caused great and beneficial changes within a generation. The more time spent in the open air the better; since however most persons who work must spend the greater part of the day indoors, ventilation is a matter of great importance.

Although fresh air enthusiasts are still too few, yet some go to the extreme and think that because cool air in motion is good, the colder the air and more violent the motion the better. On the contrary, chilling the whole body or a part of the body lowers resistance. Draughts of air have no bad effects upon persons in good health, particularly those accustomed to changes in temperature. But draughts are likely to be injurious to aged or sick persons and babies, by diminishing their resistance to such infections as common colds and pneumonia. It should be remembered that draughts or cold alone cannot cause colds; the specific germs must be present.

LIGHTING.--Amount and direction of light are physiologically important. Defects of the eyes, too prolonged use, and insufficient light are the commonest causes of eye strain. Most eye defects can be relieved by glasses. Children's eyes should be examined upon entering school, and as often afterward as the oculist advises. Prolonged use causes fatigue of the eyes, especially when the illumination is poor; within limits, the amount of light needed depends on the nature of the work. Light should come from the left side of right handed people; never from the front. Light reflected from snow, sand, glazed white paper of books, or other bright surfaces is fatiguing from its intensity, and from the unusual angle at which it enters the eyes. Too much light is harmful, and probably causes some of the effects, such as nausea and headache, commonly attributed to poor ventilation.

Almost all blindness is preventable, and blindness due to industrial accidents and processes is no exception to this rule. Surely no individual precautions or legal measures are too great in order to guard against this saddest of all physical defects.

CLEANLINESS OF HOUSES.--A clean, well-cared for house is desirable from every point of view, but certain kinds of cleanliness affect health more than others.

The most scrupulous care should be exercised wherever food is stored or prepared. The kitchen is in reality a laboratory; in it either intelligently or ignorantly are formed chemical compounds which have a far-reaching effect upon family health. From the standpoint of health no other room in the house is so important. It should be bright, airy, and easy to clean. In cleaning kitchen tables and woodwork water should not be allowed to soak into cracks and dark corners, carrying with it particles of food for the nourishment of bacteria and insects. Linoleum, if used to cover the floor, should be well fitted at the edges to prevent water from running underneath. There should be neither cracks nor crevices in wall or floor, and no dark corners or out-of-the-way cupboards in which dust, food particles, and moisture can accumulate. Such conditions not only attract mice and roaches, but furnish favorable soil for the development of moulds and fungi which by their growth affect food deleteriously. Waging a constant warfare against the development of bacteria constitutes a large part of good housekeeping.

All cooking utensils should be thoroughly washed, scalded, and dried before they are put away; the use of carelessly washed dishes is bad. Enameled or agate ware which has begun to chip should be discarded. Dish-cloths and towels should be washed and boiled after using, and if possible dried in the sun.

Every place in which food is kept should have constant care. The refrigerator is particularly important. Its linings should be water-tight, and the drain freely open at all times; otherwise the surrounding wood will become foul and saturated with drainings. At least once a week it should be entirely emptied and cleaned in the following way: The racks should be thoroughly washed in hot soapsuds to which a small amount of washing soda has been added, rinsed in boiling water, dried and placed in the sun and air. All parts of the refrigerator should be washed in the same manner, especially grooves and projections where food or dirt may lodge. The drainpipe should be flushed, the whole interior rinsed again with plain hot water, thoroughly dried with a clean cloth, and left to air for at least an hour. The drainage pan should be washed and scalded frequently. Food showing the slightest evidence of spoiling should be removed from the refrigerator at once.

Even more attention should be paid to the hands of the cook. They should be washed always before handling food, and always after visiting the toilet, using the handkerchief, or otherwise coming in contact with nose, mouth, or other bodily secretions. Theoretically coughing and sneezing ought not to occur in the neighborhood of food, especially of food to be eaten raw; and persons with coughs, colds, or other communicable disease, however slight, ought not to handle food.

If this rule were observed in practice, more persons would go hungry, but fewer would be sick.

Thorough cleaning of rooms involves soap, water, sunshine, air, and elbow grease, just as it did before germs were discovered. Cleaning means actually removing dirt and dust, not merely stirring it up to settle again; consequently dry sweeping and dusting are ineffectual. Vacuum cleaning, and sweeping and dusting with damp or "dustless" mops and dusters are good. Deodorants and disinfectants do not take the place of ordinary cleanliness.

Dust does not carry living disease germs to an appreciable extent; the fact is now well established that diseases formerly thought to be transmitted by dust or even supposed to travel directly through the air, are carried on tiny particles of moisture and mucus expelled in coughing and sneezing. This mode of transmission is called droplet or spray infection; it is one of the most active agents in spreading certain kinds of communicable diseases.

Nevertheless dust in motion is harmful; it irritates the lining membranes of the nose, throat, bronchial tubes, and lungs, even causing tiny wounds through which disease germs enter. Thus tuberculosis is especially prevalent among stone cutters, felt workers, and others engaged in dusty trades. Metallic dust is especially harmful, because it is harder and sharper than dust from organic substances like wool and cotton. Furthermore, presence of dust indicates a low standard of cleanliness. People who tolerate it generally tolerate uncleanliness in other forms, more serious though less apparent.

Cleaning would not be so great a problem if most houses were not littered with such dust catchers as carpets, so-called ornaments, carved and upholstered furniture, banners, draperies, and a vast collection of articles that can only be classified as Christmas presents. In actual practice things that are difficult or expensive to clean seldom are cleaned; carpets for example are considered unhygienic, not because they cannot be cleaned, but because they are not. William Morris' advice to exclude from houses all articles not known to be useful or believed to be beautiful would, if followed, add years to the lives of housekeepers.

GARBAGE, has little bearing on health, except in so far as it affords a breeding place for flies. If it contains disease germs it may be dangerous, but statistics show that garbage handlers, although they can hardly be called especially careful, are not more subject to sickness than other men of their class. Garbage disposal is chiefly a question of preventing a public nuisance; it is a matter of cleanliness and public decency.

INSECTS.--Flies, cockroaches, and other scavenging insects may carry disease germs on their feet and thus infect food on which they walk. Typhoid, cholera, dysentery, and other diseases have been carried by flies. Flies are always a menace, and should not be tolerated; moreover, the thought of their coming to food directly from manure piles and privy vaults is disgusting. Houses should be thoroughly screened in the fly season, but it is better to destroy the nuisance at its source. The chief breeding places of flies are garbage cans and manure piles. If the garbage can is water tight, closely covered, frequently emptied, and thoroughly cleaned, flies will not develop in it; about ten days must elapse from the time when the egg is laid until the insect is ready to fly. Fly traps to fit on the garbage can are useful. Manure should be screened and removed frequently, or it can be treated chemically. Methods for treating it are given in "Preventive Medicine and Hygiene."--Rosenau, p. 255, and in Bulletin No. 118, of the U. S. Dept. of Agriculture, July 14, 1914.

[Illustration: FIG. 8.--A FLY WITH GERMS (GREATLY MAGNIFIED) ON ITS LEGS. (*U. S. Dept. Agri.*)]

Other diseases carried by insects are malaria and yellow fever, each by a special species of mosquito; typhus fever, by lice; and bubonic plague, by rat fleas. Various diseases less common in this country are carried by other insects. Even when mosquitoes are not carrying disease germs their bites may be harmful since they are often rubbed, especially by children, until the skin is broken, and various infections may enter through the wounds. Insects of every kind, rats, mice, and vermin should be excluded from houses.

SEWAGE.--Discharges from the bowels and bladder contain various germs, and constitute one of the most important routes by which germs of typhoid fever, cholera and certain other diseases travel from person to person. Keeping sewage out of the water supply is consequently of great importance. Where a system of sewage disposal exists, the responsibility of making the system adequate and thus safeguarding public health rests upon the community as a whole. Communities ordinarily get just as much, or just as little typhoid fever as they are willing to endure.

[Illustration: FIG. 9.--HOW A WELL MAY BE POLLUTED. (*From "The Human Mechanism."* Copyright by Theodore Hough and William T. Sedgwick. Ginn and Company, publishers. Used by permission.)]

In places having no system of drainage privies must be used. They can be made harmless, as army camps prove, but they require scrupulous care. Fecal matter must be prevented from draining into wells and other water supplies, and must be screened from flies. The privy should be located at a distance from the well. The minimum distance that is safe depends in each case upon the nature of the soil and the direction of the natural drainage. Even when the privy is situated below the well on sloping ground, drainage may still occur from the privy to the well; however, a well-made, properly located pit privy is safe unless it is near a limestone formation. The dry earth system is satisfactory in places having an efficient public scavenger system; in this system pails or cans are used to receive the discharges, which are then covered with sand, ashes, earth or, preferably, chloride of lime. The buckets are frequently emptied and the contents buried at least one foot below the surface of the ground. The objection to this method for more extended use is that proper care of the cans is a disagreeable duty of which most households soon tire.

PERSONAL CLEANLINESS.--The main functions of the skin are three: to protect underlying tissues, to excrete waste matter, and to regulate bodily heat by checking or allowing the evaporation of perspiration. After perspiration has evaporated solid matter is left upon the skin, and oily matter also is deposited on it by the glands that keep the skin lubricated. Removing these and other materials at least once a day is desirable to improve the bodily tone and sense of well-being. Real cleanliness is impossible without frequent use of warm water and soap.

Cold baths are stimulating, though not very efficacious for cleansing purposes. They are valuable tonics if properly used, but delicate or elderly persons should use them only by a physician's advice. Chilly feelings or depression following should be the signal for any person to discontinue cold bathing or swimming in cold water.

Warm baths are soothing in their effects, and are appropriate at bed time, particularly for persons inclined to sleeplessness. Very hot baths, especially if prolonged, may be harmful, and should not be taken often.

There is no clear connection between general cleanliness and disease. Frequent bathing does not protect a person from any particular disease, except in so far as bathing necessarily includes washing the hands. If typhoid germs for example have actually been swallowed, a clean bodily exterior is of no avail in preventing typhoid fever or in diminishing its severity. The same is true of other diseases.

But it is impossible to emphasize unduly the importance of clean hands. Hands are prime offenders in distributing fresh bodily secretions, and germs both innocent and harmful. All health authorities agree on this point.

"Perhaps 90% of all infections are taken into the body through the mouth. They reach the mouth in water, food, fingers, dust, and upon the innumerable objects that are sometimes placed in the mouth. The fact that the great majority of infections are taken by way of the mouth gives scientific direction to personal hygiene. Sanitary habits demand that the hands should be washed after defecation and again before eating, and fingers should be kept away from the mouth and nose, and that no unnecessary objects should be mouthed. All food and drink should be clean or thoroughly cooked. These simple precautions alone would prevent many a case of infection."--(Rosenau: Preventive Medicine and Hygiene, p. 366.)

As Dr. Chapin says:

"Probably the chief vehicle for the conveyance of nasal and oral secretion from one to another is the fingers. If one takes the trouble to watch for a short time his neighbors, or even himself, unless he has been particularly trained in such matters, he will be surprised to note the number of times that the fingers go to the mouth and the nose. Not only is the saliva made use of for a great variety of purposes, and numberless articles are for one reason or another placed in the mouth, but for no reason whatever, and all unconsciously, the fingers are with great frequency raised to the lips or the nose. Who can doubt that if the salivary glands secreted indigo the fingers would continually be stained a deep blue, and who can doubt that if the nasal and oral secretions contain the germs of disease these germs will be almost as constantly found upon the fingers? All successful commerce is reciprocal, and in this universal trade in human saliva the fingers not only bring foreign secretions to the mouth of their owner, but there exchanging them for his own, distribute the latter to everything that the hand touches. This happens not once, but scores and hundreds of times during the day's round of the individual. The cook spreads his saliva on the muffins and rolls, the waitress infects the glasses and spoons, the moistened fingers of the peddler arrange his fruit, the thumb of the milkman is in his measure, the reader moistens the pages of his book, the conductor his transfer tickets, the "lady" the fingers of her glove. Every one is busily engaged in this distribution of saliva, so that the end of each day finds this secretion freely distributed on the doors, window sills, furniture and playthings in the home, the straps of trolley cars, the rails and counter and desks of shops and public buildings, and indeed upon everything that the hands of man touch. What avails it if the pathogens do die quickly? A fresh supply is furnished each day."--(Chapin: The Sources and Modes of Infection, p. 188.)

ORAL HYGIENE.--Cleanliness and proper care of the mouth and teeth can hardly be over emphasized. Their bearing upon health is direct. Long ago it was recognized that persons with decayed or missing teeth frequently suffered from dyspepsia, a natural result of inability to masticate properly, but only within recent years has it been realized that decayed teeth give rise to many other diseased conditions. Bacteria are constantly present in the mouth. If the mucus of the mouth is not removed, it forms a sticky coat upon the surfaces of the teeth and gums. In this bacteria collect, and pus or matter may also be formed, which, if carried by the blood to other parts of the body, may cause digestive troubles, rheumatism, and diseases of heart and kidneys. (See Dr. T. B. Hartzell, Health News, Oct., 1915, "The Importance of Mouth Hygiene and How to Practise it.")

To keep the mouth and teeth healthy they must have:

1. Proper use.

2. Proper care.

3. Proper treatment.

1. Teeth, like other parts of the body, need exercise. Foods that require a considerable amount of chewing should be included in the diet. Such food is needed by children as soon as their first teeth have come, but care must be exercised to see that the food is actually chewed before it is swallowed.

2. A good brush should be provided. The stiffness of the bristles should be regulated according to the individual. The brush should be thoroughly rinsed after using, and discarded as soon as it is worn. Dental floss is generally needed to remove particles that have lodged between the teeth.

Brushing the teeth by passing the bristles across them is not efficacious. They should be brushed not across but with the cracks, as a good housewife sweeps a floor.

"In the light of recent investigation conducted by some of the leading students of mouth hygiene, the most effective way to use the toothbrush is to place the bristles of the brush firmly against the teeth, applying firm pressure, as though trying to force the bristles between the teeth, using a slight rotary or scrubbing motion.... After a little practice the user of this method will be surprised at the results obtained. Care should be used to go over all the surfaces of the teeth in this manner."--(See Dr. W. G. Ebersole. "The Importance of Mouth Hygiene and How to Practice it," Health News, Oct., 1915.)

After brushing the teeth, the mouth should be rinsed by forcing lukewarm water about the teeth, using all the force that can be brought to bear by the cheeks, lips, and tongue.

3. TREATMENT.--The teeth, including the first teeth of children, should be inspected by a competent dentist at least twice a year. Periodic cleansing by a dentist, and early attention to small cavities, may prevent serious ill health and impairment of the body, as well as the acute suffering generally accompanying treatment of advanced dental defects.

CLOTHING.--Clothing was originally used for purposes of ornament. Desire for protection from cold and dampness came later. The amount of clothing required varies greatly according to individual needs and habits, but it is increasingly recognized that light clothing is best, provided that the wearer is really protected from cold. Clothing should be porous in order to allow ventilation of the body, supported so far as possible from the shoulders, and clean and well aired. Dampness favors the growth of germs which may cause irritation of the skin.

Clothing should not constrict the body or hamper its movements. Perhaps the worst health menace for which clothing is to blame comes from the high heeled shoes on which many women prefer to limp through life. From the health standpoint shoes are of great importance. Bad shoes are responsible for many cases of flat feet, whose muscles have degenerated through non-use, and for much so-called "rheumatism," which is merely the protest of abused muscles. Bad shoes also, by distorting the feet, prevent comfortable walking, which is the only out-of-door exercise readily available for the vast majority of people; and still worse, the resulting unnatural position of the body sometimes has serious consequences by bringing injurious strains on other muscles and organs.

FOOD.--Two distinct problems are encountered here: the problem of nutrition, and the problem of preventing sickness. Nutrition, or proper feeding, is a subject beyond the scope of this book; it is nevertheless one of the most important, if not the most important, factor in maintaining health. Food preparation and care of children, the two most important functions of the home, are unfortunately relegated to the least intelligent and least interested members of most households in which servants are employed.

Most American families eat too much protein food, such as meat and eggs. Excess of protein probably leads to degeneration of tissues, and plays a part in causing the degenerative diseases already mentioned. Habit is important here as in other ways of living, but cereals and vegetables should in large measure make up the diet of sedentary persons and indeed of everyone in warm weather.

The amount of food required in 24 hours depends on many factors: age, height, weight, occupation, season, and habit. Underweight and overweight are both abnormal conditions; probably the latter is the more easily remedied. Both require the advice of a physician. Rapid reduction of weight involves certain dangers, especially for persons with weak hearts.

Food may cause sickness either because it is in itself harmful, or because it carries disease germs. Meat from diseased animals should be destroyed before it reaches the market, but bacterial activities in food originally wholesome may form in it poisonous substances.

The chief diseases known to be carried by food, water, or milk are typhoid fever, paratyphoid, dysentery and other diarrhoeal diseases, scarlet fever, diphtheria, septic sore throat, and tuberculosis. The sole problem here is to keep human and animal excretions out of food, water, and milk. Since thorough cooking kills disease germs, danger arises chiefly from raw foods. All fruits and vegetables eaten raw should first be thoroughly washed.

Water is essential to health. At least three pints should be taken daily, the amount varying somewhat according to diet, exercise, temperature, and so forth. Most persons drink too little water.

Cities and towns should of course have public supplies of pure water. Contamination of water, when it occurs, is caused chiefly by sewage from cesspools, privies, and drains. All well or spring water must be constantly watched and Boards of Health are always ready to examine samples of water and to report whether it is safe to drink. At the present time a porcelain filter is the only satisfactory kind for a household, but many domestic filters are so badly cared for that in actual practice they are worse than none. Danger from a filter containing an accumulation of impurities is greater than the danger from most ordinary water supplies. Boiling water for ten minutes kills all pathogenic germs, but this method is inconvenient on a large scale and is not practical for continued family use.

Every effort should be made to insure a regular supply of pure water in every house. It is not satisfactory to have two kinds, one for drinking and one for other purposes, since mistakes are sure to be made, especially by children. Some families who use only bottled or filtered water for drinking purposes habitually run the risk involved in using impure water from the tap for cleaning the teeth.

Freezing destroys most germs, but ice is not necessarily free from bacterial life, and should be used in drinking water only when known to be free from impurities. Neither does freezing milk or cream necessarily kill germs that may be contained in it.

Raw milk plays so important a part in the spread of disease that its fitness for human consumption is open to serious question. Certified milk, where obtainable, is safe but expensive. Boiled milk is safe, but changed in taste and to some extent in quality. If milk is heated to 142°-145° F. and kept at that temperature for 30 minutes all disease germs in it are killed. This process, called pasteurization, renders milk safe. The objection is sometimes made that continued use of pasteurized milk for infants causes scurvy, but in New York City where over 90 per cent. of the milk is pasteurized no increase in scurvy has been noticed, while a large diminution in deaths of infants from diarrhoeal diseases has resulted, as in all cities where pasteurization is required.

The following is a simple method for pasteurizing a quart bottle of milk. If the directions are exactly followed the milk will be pasteurized at the end of the process; no thermometer need be used. To prevent the bottle from breaking, it is first warmed by placing it for a few minutes in a pail of warm water.

"From the results of the experiments it was concluded that any housewife can pasteurize a one quart bottle of milk by:

1. Boiling 2½ quarts of water in a large agate saucepan; or better

2. Boiling 2 quarts of water in a 10 pound tin lard pail, placing the slightly warmed bottle from the ice chest in it, covering with a cloth and setting in a warm place. At the end of one hour the bottle of milk should be removed and chilled promptly. The water must be boiled in the container in which the pasteurization is to be done."--(Ruth Vories, in "Health News," Sept., 1916.)

ELIMINATION.--Careful attention should be paid to elimination through the bowels and kidneys. Constipation is responsible for many common ailments; among them are headache, disinclination to work, irritable temper, and lowered resistance. If long continued, constipation becomes serious both from congestion and displacement of pelvic organs, and from absorption over a considerable time of even small amounts of the poisonous substances resulting from decomposition of food in the large intestine. The bowels can best be regulated by diet, water, exercise, and habit. The habitual use of cathartic and laxative drugs is most unwise, because they tend to aggravate the trouble. Moreover the habitual and continued use of injections and "internal baths" is harmful, and would not be considered necessary if bran and coarse flour and vegetables were substituted for concentrated foods. Greed, laziness, and lack of intelligence lead most persons suffering with constipation to prefer pills to the restraints demanded by hygienic living. The habit of evacuating the bowels at a regular time, if established in early childhood and rigidly adhered to, will prevent constipation among most healthy people. Any person who thinks drugs necessary should consult a physician, and be prepared to follow the régime he advises over a considerable period of time and at the cost of some self-denial.

For healthy people, voiding urine presents no difficulty if a sufficient amount of water is taken; but some persons reduce the amount of liquid taken in order to escape the inconvenience of urination. This practice is harmful, and may involve insufficient cleansing of the entire system. If frequent urination disturbs sleep, liquids may be withheld during the evening; but the total amount of water taken in 24 hours should not be diminished.

REST AND FATIGUE.--A fatigued person is a poisoned person. Muscular exertion burns the fuel constituents of the body, as we recognize by the greater heat generated within us during muscular exertion. Waste products, resulting from this burning process, accumulate if not removed, and clog the body in somewhat the same way that ashes and cinders clog a furnace. The fatigued person remains fatigued, consequently, until the accumulations of waste matter are removed by the normal action of the lungs, skin, and kidneys.

Fatigue is caused by both mental and physical work, and when excessive, affects the nervous system most disastrously. The body can and should respond to occasional extra drafts on strength and endurance; its flexibility and power of adjusting to varying conditions may even be stimulated thereby. But even slight fatigue, if continued and especially if associated with anxiety or worry, has caused many nervous and mental breakdowns.

Work carried beyond the point of normal fatigue requires a proportionately longer time for recovery. For example, if the point of fatigue has been reached by a certain finger muscle after 15 contractions, and if half an hour is required to rest it completely, one might suppose that one hour would rest it after 30 contractions. This is not so, however; after 30 contractions 2 hours are required, or 4 times as much rest for twice the amount of work, if continued beyond the point of fatigue. Laboratory experiments and experience alike show that this principle holds true in other forms of fatigue. Thus the output of factories has been shown in many instances to be greater, other things being equal, when operatives work 8 hours a day than when they work longer. Excessive hours in any kind of work are the poorest economy.

Fatigue is increased in direct proportion not only to muscular exertion but also to the amount of speed, complexity, responsibility, monotony, noise, and confusion involved in an occupation. Ability to bear fatigue differs greatly with different people, as ability varies to bear other kinds of strain. Rest at night and on Sunday, and the annual vacation should be enough to keep a person in good condition. If not, there is probably something wrong with the worker's health, the nature of his work, or his adaptation to his particular kind of work. This statement is not only true of persons regularly employed, but of those living at home, including children in school, women in "society," and especially mothers of families.

SLEEP.--A sufficient amount of sleep is essential to health, but individual requirements vary widely. Each person should know and regard his own need, and children and young people should be obliged to go to bed early. Ability to sleep is largely habit; good habits should be formed and continued. Sleep-producing drugs should never be taken, except by a doctor's prescription.

RECREATION.--Owing to the speed, complexity, and worry of modern life among all classes, and to the monotony of work in industry, recreation has become a matter of vital importance for everyone. Some muscular activity, preferably in the open air, is needed by every healthy person. Recreation should be as unlike the regular occupation as possible: going to the theatre, for example, is not the best exercise for sedentary workers employed all day in artificially lighted offices. The element of pleasure is essential. Hoisting dumb-bells purely from conscientious motives is seldom beneficial, and is generally soon abandoned.

The part played by habit in matters of health is often overlooked. Although the body adjusts itself to widely varying conditions and even to unfavorable ones, the importance of forming desirable habits cannot be overemphasized. Sudden or radical changes in living, however, particularly among people no longer young, may play havoc. New and violent systems of exercise, weight reduction, and food fads forced on families by enthusiastic discoverers involve considerable risk.

Many elements enter into health; in no single one is found hygienic salvation. Temptation always exists to emphasize one element at the expense of others. For instance, people who insist upon overventilating rooms regardless of others' comfort may themselves be utterly careless in regard to necessary sleep, and more than one fastidiously clean person has disregarded the highly unclean condition of constipation. To maintain sound health only a rational program will suffice: properly balanced work and play, sleep and food and all other elements must be included in due proportion. And over-anxious health seekers might well remember that health is not so much an end in itself, as a means to a happy and productive life; even in concern over health, it is possible for him that saveth his life to lose it.

EXERCISES

1. Explain the difference between an hereditary disease and hereditary susceptibility to a disease. How may hereditary susceptibility to a disease be combatted?

2. What are the essentials of good ventilation?

3. What is the proper temperature for a living room? What are the effects of higher temperatures? Of lower temperatures?

4. Describe methods for maintaining household cleanliness.

5. Discuss the importance from the point of view of health, of dust; of insects; of garbage; of sewage.

6. What principles should guide one in deciding whether a certain water supply is safe to use for drinking purposes? What are the dangers of impure water? How can impure water be rendered safe?

7. What diseases may be carried by milk? How can milk be rendered safe?

8. Explain the health aspects of personal cleanliness.

9. What care should be given the teeth and mouth? Why?

10. What bad results frequently follow constipation? How should constipation be remedied?

11. Name seven factors that are important in causing fatigue. Why is it uneconomical to continue work, either physical or mental, beyond the point of fatigue?

12. What facilities for recreation, especially in the open air, does your community provide for little children? For school children? For working boys and girls? For grown people?

FOR FURTHER READING

Health and Disease--Roger I. Lee, Introduction and Chapters I, III-V, VII-IX.

How to Live--Fisher and Fisk, Chapters I, III-V.

The Human Mechanism--Hough and Sedgwick, Chapters V, XXII-XXIX.

Disease and Its Causes--Councilman, Chapters X, XII.

Fatigue and Efficiency--Goldmark, Chapters II, III.

Preventive Medicine and Hygiene--Rosenau.

A Manual of Personal Hygiene--6th Edition, Edited by Walter L. Pyle.

Four Epochs of a Woman's Life--Galbraith.

Hygiene and Physical Culture for Women--Galbraith.

The Home and Its Management--Kittredge.

Exercise and Health--F. C. Smith, Supplement 24 to the Public Health Reports, Government Printing Office, Washington.

The Sanitary Privy--Farmers' Bulletin 463, United States Department of Agriculture, Government Printing Office, Washington.

Safe Disposal of Human Excreta at Unsewered Homes--Lumsden, Stiles and Freeman, Bulletin 68, Public Health Reports, Government Printing Office, Washington.

The Disposal of Human Excreta and Sewage of the Country Home--New York State Department of Health, Albany.

Milk and Its Relation to Public Health--Bulletin 56, Hygienic Laboratory, Government Printing Office, Washington.

Milk and Its Relation to Health--New York State Department of Health, Albany.

Other Publications of the United States Public Health Service and of the Departments of Health of the different states and cities.

CHAPTER III

BABIES AND THEIR CARE

The principles of hygiene are fundamentally the same for young and old. The applications, however, differ at different ages. From the time when physical growth and development are complete until changes due to old age appear, an individual commonly has greater resistance than at other ages, and is able in consequence to endure unfavorable conditions of life with more success.

Babies, on the other hand, are exceedingly sensitive to their environment. Surroundings that are even slightly unfavorable are likely to make babies sick. In order to remain healthy, they must have exactly the right kind of food, in the right quantities and at the right times; their sleep, exercise, and clothing must be carefully regulated; they must be protected from careless handling, from nervous strain, and above all, from the many kinds of infection to which they are peculiarly susceptible. The life of a baby fortunately can be controlled almost completely; when properly regulated it offers, therefore, an unequalled opportunity to see how hygienic principles work out in actual practice.

The primitive mother's instinct to nourish and protect and succor her helpless child was the original form of nursing. Instinct alone, unfortunately, has never accomplished much in preserving health. The human race has now had an experience in the care of infants that extends over thousands of years. Yet today we are still, on the whole, less successful in keeping babies alive than we are in raising domestic animals; we still allow society to continue, like a modern Herod, in its ruthless career of slaughtering the innocents.

About 14 babies out of every 100 born in the registration area[1] of the United States die before reaching the age of one year, while in some of our industrial cities as many as 25 out of every 100 born die before they are a year old. Most of these deaths are preventable. Thus, in a few American cities, the death rates have been so reduced that fewer than 10 babies out of every 100 die before completing the first year; while in Dunedin, New Zealand, as a result of the work of the Society for the Health of Women and Children, the infant death rate has been so reduced that in 1912 only about 4 out of every 100 babies died before they were a year old.

While ignorant mothers, who may or may not be uneducated women, and contaminated milk, are as a matter of fact, chiefly responsible for our high infant death rates, yet as we have already seen, every factor in the environment has its effect upon a baby. This fact has led Sir Arthur Newsholme, an eminent English authority, to say:

"Infant Mortality is the most sensitive index we possess of social welfare. If babies were well born and well cared for, their mortality would be negligible. The infant death rate measures the intelligence, health, and right living of fathers and mothers, the standards of morals and sanitation of communities and governments, the efficiency of physicians, nurses, health officers, and educators."

Care of the child should begin at the earliest possible moment: that is, nearly nine months before he is born. Care before birth, for want of a better name, is called prenatal care of the mother. Every woman who thinks that she is pregnant should put herself at once under the care of a competent physician, so that he can make the necessary examinations as early as possible. If she follows his advice in regard to hygiene and proper regulation of her life, she may be free from anxiety, and may justly expect that her delivery will be a safe and normal process.

A demonstration of the value of prenatal care was recently made by the Boston District Nursing Association. During the year 1915 prenatal care was given to 751 expectant mothers in 5 wards of the city; each woman attended a pregnancy clinic, where she was under the care of an experienced obstetrician, and was visited at intervals by a nurse who kept careful watch of her general condition and gave necessary advice and encouragement. In consequence the death rate among the babies whose mothers had prenatal care was only half as great, through the whole first year of life, as the death rate of babies in the same wards whose mothers had not had prenatal care. Moreover, the rate of still-births was only half as great as the rate among the general population of Boston. If prenatal care can save so many lives, surely it ought to be available for every pregnant woman in the land, including even that generally neglected class of people who are neither very rich nor very poor.

Each baby's birth should be recorded by the registrar of births, and parents should make sure that registration has been attended to in the city or town where they live. In some states birth registration is already obligatory, but in any case it is required by the child's own interest. For instance, in later life it may be necessary for him to prove the date and place of birth in order to establish, among other things, his right to vote and to inherit property, and to settle the question of his liability to military service. Moreover, complete and accurate birth registration is needed by every community because it is essential to such reforms as reducing infant mortality and abolishing child labor.

GROWTH AND DEVELOPMENT

Statements in regard to growth and development are based on observations of many children. It should be remembered that the following figures represent averages only, and that healthy children may vary from them considerably without giving cause for alarm.

AVERAGE SIZE.--The average weight of a baby at birth is from 7 to 7½ lbs. and the average length is about 20 inches, but it is not unusual for a child to weigh anywhere from 5 to 10 pounds at birth and to measure from 16 to 22 inches in length. During the first week of life a baby loses slightly in weight. After the first week a healthy baby should gain from 4 to 8 ounces a week until he is six months old; after that time the weekly gain is less. The weight at birth will usually double during the first five months, and treble during the first year. Consequently, a baby weighing 7 pounds at birth may be expected to weigh 14 pounds when five months old, and 21 pounds when a year old. Weight is one of the most important indications of a baby's condition. He should be weighed every week during the first 6 months, once in two weeks during the second 6 months, and once a month throughout the 2nd year.

MUSCULAR DEVELOPMENT.--A baby at birth is helpless, and during the first few months he has little muscular control. During the third month he ordinarily begins to lift his head, and he can usually hold it up without support by the time he is 3 months old; when 7 to 8 months old he sits erect and begins to play with toys. From this time a baby makes rapid progress; he attempts to stand on his feet, begins to creep, and by the time he is 14 months old he is usually able to stand alone, or even to walk a few steps. He is usually running about without difficulty when fifteen or sixteen months old.

Babies should never be urged to walk or to bear their weight on their feet. If healthy they are generally eager to go about unaided, and like to investigate their surroundings without assistance. If walking is unusually delayed, a physician should be consulted.

DEVELOPMENT OF SPECIAL SENSES.--A new-born baby is unable to distinguish objects, but the eyes are sensitive to light and need careful protection. Hearing, although undeveloped at birth, soon becomes acute; consequently the child should stay in a quiet room. When six or eight weeks old he notices objects, and at three months old he welcomes his mother when he is hungry. A month or two later he begins to distinguish between familiar and unfamiliar faces, and to show approval or disapproval.

DEVELOPMENT OF SPEECH.--A baby six or seven months old begins consciously to utter sounds, and usually can say a few unconnected words by the time he is a year old. The average child, however, does not begin to form sentences of more than two or three words until he is about two years old.

DEVELOPMENT OF TEETH.--The so-called milk teeth are twenty in number; they are followed by thirty-two permanent teeth. The two lower front teeth (central incisors) generally appear when a child is from five to nine months old, and in from one to three months later the four upper front teeth (upper incisors) appear. All the first or milk teeth should have come through by the time a child is two and a half years old, but wide variations occur both in the time and order of appearance and should occasion no uneasiness if the child seems well. Unusual conditions of any sort should be referred to the physician; it is a great mistake to attribute all illness at this time to teething.

The first of the permanent teeth appear when a child is about six years old. Mothers sometimes mistake the first permanent molars for temporary teeth, a mistake that frequently leads to neglect and even extraction of highly important teeth. All but the last four molars, sometimes called wisdom teeth, should be through by the time a child is fifteen. The wisdom teeth may not appear before the 20th or even the 25th year.

NORMAL EXCRETIONS.--A new-born baby should have one or two bowel movements during the first twenty-four hours; the first bowel movements are sticky and almost black in color. After the baby begins to nurse, three to four movements a day are not unusual, and throughout infancy and childhood as well as adult life there should be one or two evacuations of the bowels daily. The character of the stools is more important than the number. While the baby is taking milk only, the movements should be soft, yellow in color, and nearly odorless. Change in frequency of the movements, or appearance of undigested food or curds of milk in the stool, should be carefully noted and if continued, reported to a physician; they may be the first signs of serious digestive trouble.

The urine of an infant should be odorless and colorless. It should be voided at least once during the first twenty-four hours, and much more frequently after the baby begins to nurse. Marked diminution in the amount of urine should be reported to a doctor.

Efforts should be made early to develop habits of regularity in the evacuation of the bladder and bowels. If taken up regularly most children learn to use a chamber for bowel movements by the time they are three months old. Normal children, if properly trained, usually have no bladder discharge during the night after they are 18 months old, and they learn even earlier to indicate a desire to urinate during the day time.

CLOTHING.--The amount and weight of a baby's clothing should depend upon the season; but garments worn next to the skin, except the diaper, should be wholly or partly of wool, the lightest weight in summer and heavier weight in winter. During the first few weeks a baby's abdomen should be supported by a flannel binder about six inches wide, applied snugly but not tightly enough to restrict either the abdomen or chest walls. It may be replaced later by a loosely fitting knitted band worn for warmth only. Such a band is especially necessary if there is tendency to diarrhoea, but in no case should it be discarded before the 18th month. All garments except the diaper and first flannel binder should hang from the shoulders, and should fit loosely but well.

Clothing for babies should be of soft materials and should be simply made. Even the first clothes should not be very long. The weight of very long clothing is an unnecessary burden, and prevents free movements of the legs. At night an entire change of clothing should be made, and a nightgown of warmer material substituted for the petticoat and slip. Most children are dressed too warmly indoors, but in low temperatures they need to be well protected.

Diapers should be soft and absorbent. It may be necessary to wash new diapers several times before using in order to make them soft enough. Care should be taken not to apply them too tightly, or in such a way as to cause pressure on the genitals. They should be changed during the day whenever wet or soiled, and at night when the baby is taken up to be fed. Proper care of diapers is highly important, however laborious. They should be well washed, boiled, and thoroughly dried before they are used a second time. Diapers that have been wet but not soiled should not be dried and used again before being washed. Much work can be saved if pads of loosely woven absorbent material are used inside the diaper to receive discharges. The pads can be burned, but even if washed the labor is less than washing full sized diapers. Like all other infant's garments, diapers should be washed with pure white soap and without starch. Waterproof material used to cover the diaper is almost sure to irritate the baby's skin, and is consequently harmful.

SLEEP.--During his first few weeks a normal baby sleeps about nine-tenths of the time, and should be left undisturbed except for necessary care. He should sleep in a crib, bassinet or basket protected from light and drafts; in no circumstances should a baby sleep in the bed with his mother or any other person. Pillows are unnecessary for babies, and indeed for older children, but if used they should be thin and firm.

The amount of sleep necessary gradually diminishes, but during all the years of growth a child needs more sleep than an adult. The amount of sleep required daily is approximately as follows:

First month 18 to 20 hours Second to sixth month 16 to 18 hours Sixth month to one year 14 to 15 hours One to two years 13 to 14 hours Two to four years 11 to 12 hours

After this time a child should sleep at least ten hours out of the twenty-four. During the first year a nap in the middle of the forenoon and another in the afternoon are desirable. A child who is inclined to sleep so long that his nap interferes with his night's sleep, should be waked from his nap, but at the same hour every day. When a child is a year old, one nap during the day is often sufficient, if he is doing well, but the habit of taking a nap at some time during the day should be continued through the fifth year if possible, or even later.

Babies should not be rocked or otherwise coaxed to go to sleep; they should be made comfortable and then left alone. They learn to go to sleep by themselves as soon as they are convinced that sleep is expected of them, and that no unfounded objections on their part will be regarded. Continued inability to sleep normally usually indicates discomfort or poor general condition, and should be taken up with the doctor. Pacifiers and thumb-sucking should not be allowed, since they lead to changes in the shape of the jaw with resulting imperfect adjustment of the teeth. Soothing syrup and like medicines should never be given to a baby; death or permanent injury has resulted from their use. It is impossible to emphasize too strongly the danger of giving them even a single time.

FRESH AIR.--All that has been said about the importance of fresh air for adults applies with even greater force to infants and children. During his first month especially a baby is susceptible to draughts; nevertheless, the room should be well ventilated and its temperature kept between 68° and 70° F. during the day, and at about 65° F. at night. Even in cold weather the room should be well aired two or three times a day; the baby should be removed to another room while the windows are open. After the baby is three or four months old the windows may be left open at night provided the outside temperature does not fall below freezing. A healthy baby two or three weeks old may be taken out-of-doors for a short time in mild weather; when he is three months old he may be taken out-of-doors even in winter on bright sunny days. The time spent out-of-doors should be gradually increased until the baby stays out the greater part of the day; but he should not be exposed to storms, wind, flying dust, dampness, extremes of temperature, or insects. The eyes should not be covered by veils, but they should be shielded from the direct rays of the sun at all times.

DIET.--A baby, in order to thrive, must have suitable food, given at regular intervals. During the first few months of life no other food can take the place of mother's milk. Breast-fed babies are more robust than bottle-fed babies; more than this, they are less likely to contract infectious diseases or to suffer from digestive disorders. The number of bottle-fed babies who die every year is three times as great as the number of breast-fed babies who die. Many mothers do not understand the risk involved in weaning small babies; and so every year many little lives are lost, and lost needlessly. When poverty forces nursing mothers to wean their babies and seek work outside their homes, one can only say that a society which tolerates such a waste of infant life is indeed regardless of its own welfare.

Special conditions, of course, may make it undesirable for a mother to nurse her baby. No one but the physician is competent to decide this; not even neighbors, grandmothers, other members of the family, or the mother herself. Where artificial feeding must be used, it should be carefully adapted to the individual child, and in consequence it must be prescribed by the doctor. Patent foods, notwithstanding the claims on their printed labels, should be used only under his advice.

INTERVALS OF FEEDING.--Little milk is secreted during the first two days after the birth of a child. The baby should, nevertheless, be put to the breast as soon as he has had his first bath, if the mother is sufficiently rested. Always before and after nursing the mother's nipples should be washed in water that has been boiled. Nursing should be repeated at intervals of six hours during the first two days.

The following schedule for the feeding of healthy babies is given by Holt in "Care and Feeding of Infants." (1917.)

SCHEDULE FOR HEALTHY INFANTS FOR THE FIRST YEAR

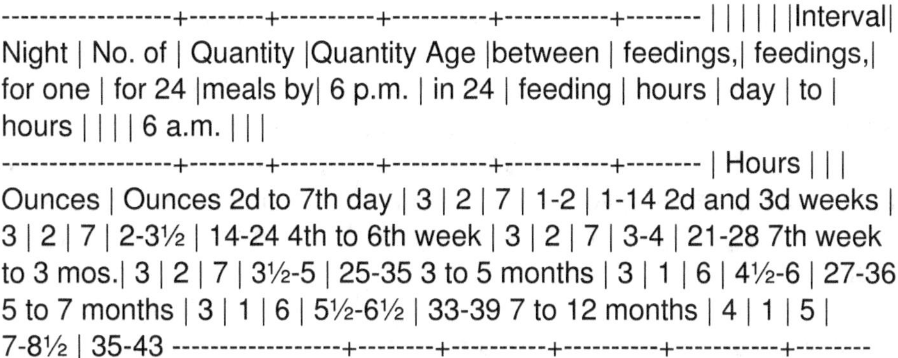

Age	Interval between feeding, Hours	Night feedings, 6 p.m. to 6 a.m.	No. of feedings in 24 hours	Quantity for one meal, Ounces	Quantity for 24 hours, Ounces
2d to 7th day	3	2	7	1-2	1-14
2d and 3d weeks	3	2	7	2-3½	14-24
4th to 6th week	3	2	7	3-4	21-28
7th week to 3 mos.	3	2	7	3½-5	25-35
3 to 5 months	3	1	6	4½-6	27-36
5 to 7 months	3	1	6	5½-6½	33-39
7 to 12 months	4	1	5	7-8½	35-43

During the period when seven feedings are given in 24 hours the following hours will be found convenient: 6 a.m., 9 a.m., 12 m., 3 p.m., 6 p.m., 10 p.m. and 2 a.m. The 2 a.m. feeding is the one omitted when the number of feedings is reduced from seven to six. Food should be given on exact schedule time; the baby if asleep should be waked for any meal except the one due at 2 a.m.

WATER.--Pure boiled water should be given regularly even to a young baby. He is often satisfied with a little warm water if he is fretful between the hours of nursing. Water may be given from a cup, a spoon, or a bottle; it is desirable, however, for the baby to learn to drink from a cup before the period of weaning begins.

WEANING.--Ordinarily, a baby should be fed from the breast until he is seven months old, either exclusively or with the exception after the second month of one bottle-feeding in twenty-four hours. This exception will do the baby no harm and may be a great relief to his mother. Partial breast-feeding should continue if possible through the ninth month, but every baby should be entirely weaned by the time he is one year old. It may be necessary, if either the baby or the mother is not thriving, to change the food before the ninth month; but it is desirable not to make the change in hot weather. Healthy babies, it should be remembered, increase in weight constantly, and steady gain in weight is the best indication that a baby's food is suitable.

NURSING BOTTLES AND NIPPLES.--Nursing bottles should be of heavy glass, cylindrical in shape, without angles or corners to make cleaning difficult. The number of bottles provided should be two or three more than the number of feedings given in 24 hours.

Short black rubber nipples which slip over the neck of the bottles should be selected. They should be of such a shape that they can easily be turned inside out; a nipple turner costs little, and is well worth the price. Nipples should be discarded when they become soft or when the opening grows so large that the milk runs in a stream rather than drop by drop.

As soon as the baby has finished his meal, the bottle should be removed from his mouth, rinsed in clear hot water, and left standing filled with cold water until a convenient time for boiling all the bottles to be used during the next 24 hours. Sufficient time must be allowed for the bottles to cool thoroughly between the time when they are boiled and the time when they are refilled. When it is time to boil the bottles they should be placed in an agate or other suitable kettle, covered with water, and boiled vigorously for three minutes. A cloth placed in the bottom of the kettle will help to prevent the bottles from breaking. After the bottles have been removed from the boiling water, they should be stoppered at once, either with rubber stoppers or plugs of sterile cotton. The stoppers, if used, should be boiled with the bottles; sterile cotton may be purchased by the package.

An easy and satisfactory method to care for rubber nipples is the following: Provide as many nipples as the number of feedings given in 24 hours, and another, if desired, to be used in case of accident; provide also two cups of ordinary white enamel, each one large enough to hold all the nipples at once. One cup should have a cover; the other should not. To avoid mistakes it is well to have the cups different in shape. As soon as each feeding is finished the nipple should be thoroughly cleansed under running water by scrubbing it inside and out with a nipple brush. The nipple thus cleansed is placed in the cup without a cover. When all the nipples have been used, cleansed, and collected in the uncovered cup, they are transferred into the other cup; water is added, the cup is covered and its contents are boiled for three minutes. The nipples remain covered in the boiled water until needed; they are removed one by one for the successive feedings. Care must be used in removing a nipple to take it by the rim, not to touch other nipples during the process and not to dip the fingers into the water. The best way is to remove them by means of a glass rod, which is boiled with the nipples and kept with them in the cup when not in use. There are several advantages of this method of caring for nipples: it is easy; it reduces to a minimum the necessary handling of the nipples after boiling; and it reduces the probability of using the wrong nipple, since boiled nipples are always in one kind of receptacle and used nipples in another. It also prevents the too common practice of continuing to keep nipples in a supposedly antiseptic solution long after the solution has become badly soiled.

TABLES of diet for children over one year of age may be found in the Appendix, page 322.

BATHING.--Usually the cord has separated and the navel has entirely healed by the time a baby is 10 days old. After this time a daily tub bath should be given; it should be given not less than one hour after feeding. The temperature of the room should be from 70-72°, measured by a thermometer placed in the part of the room where the bath is to take place. In order to avoid chilling or tiring the baby the bath should be given quickly, without confusion or interruption; success can be achieved by using even a moderate amount of foresight. Before undressing the baby everything to be used should be collected and placed within easy reach,--clean clothing, soft towels, 2 wash cloths, pure white soap, powder, absorbent cotton, etc. The bath tub should last of all be filled with water, and its temperature tested by means of a bath thermometer. The temperature of the water should be from 98° to 100°. After the baby is three months old slightly cooler water should be splashed over his chest, back, neck, and arms just after he is removed from the tub, and as he grows older the temperature of his cool splash can be reduced. Children who become accustomed to cool water in this way take kindly to their cold showers later.

The baby's face should be washed first and dried carefully, while his body is still covered. Next the head should be washed; a little soap should be used, but it must on no account enter the eyes. Next the entire body should be soaped with the hand; and then the baby should be placed gently in the bath, his head and shoulders supported by the attendant's left hand and forearm. Care should be taken to rinse off all the soap. The baby should not stay in the tub more than 2 or 3 minutes; after he has been removed from the tub he should be wrapped at once in a soft bath towel. He should be dried gently but thoroughly by patting with soft, warm towels rather than by rubbing. Folds of the skin should be dried with special care. A little powder may be applied, but a baby who is kept both clean and dry will not need much powder, if any. The baby should next be quickly dressed, with as little turning and moving as possible. Clothing should be drawn on over the feet instead of over the head, and the petticoat should be placed inside the slip so that the two garments may go on simultaneously.

EYES.--Secretion accumulating in the corners of a baby's eyes should be removed by means of a bit of absorbent cotton moistened in boiled water. The secretion should be wiped away gently; a different piece of cotton should be used for each eye, and a piece that has been used should not be put back into the water. Further than this, eyes in a normal condition do not need cleansing.

Every person who handles a baby should be very sure that her hands are clean; she should be doubly sure before she touches his eyes, since a baby's eyes are peculiarly susceptible to infection from any source. More than a quarter of all totally blind persons in the United States became blind by infection of the eyes at birth. Blindness of the new born can be prevented in practically all cases if the doctor uses a preparation of silver in the baby's eyes immediately after birth. This treatment is effective and entirely safe.

If at any time the eyelids look red or swollen, or if a drop of matter appears between the lids, the physician should be summoned at once. Total blindness may result if treatment is delayed even a few hours.

MOUTH.--The mouth should be rinsed after feeding by giving the baby a teaspoonful of boiled water. Until the teeth come it does not require other cleansing, and attempts to clean it may injure the delicate membranes that line it. Indeed, except in an emergency, fingers should not be inserted into a baby's mouth. The teeth when they appear should be cleaned by means of a soft tooth-brush.

NOSTRILS.--The nostrils need no cleaning other than removal of mucus that can easily be reached by means of a piece of cotton. If a little vaseline is placed in the nostrils on a small piece of absorbent cotton in the early morning, collections of mucus will usually be softened so that they can be removed easily at bath time.

GENITAL ORGANS.--The genital organs of girl babies should be gently washed twice a day, using absorbent cotton, and tepid water. Treatment other than cleanliness is ordinarily unnecessary. Vaseline may be applied if the genitals are slightly reddened; any discharge or abnormal appearance should be reported to the doctor. In the case of boy babies the foreskin should be gently drawn back twice a week after immersion in the tub; after the parts have been gently washed with absorbent cotton, it should be drawn forward again. No force should be employed in retracting the foreskin; the physician should be consulted if it cannot be retracted easily.

THE DEVELOPMENT OF HABITS.--During his first few months crying is a child's only means of expression, and he quickly learns to make effective use of his limited opportunities. It is important for the mother to distinguish between crying caused by pain, illness, or hunger, and crying caused by temper. These cries are more or less distinctive, but no one can be sure in every case just what a crying baby is attempting to express.

A cry caused by hunger is fretful and often interrupted by sucking the thumb; it ceases when the child is fed. A cry caused by indigestion is similar; the child is relieved for a short time by feeding, but soon begins to cry again. If he has acute pain, such as earache, the cry is sharp, repeated at frequent intervals and accompanied by other symptoms of distress, such as restlessness, contraction of the features, and drawing up the legs. In serious illness the cry is usually feeble, fairly constant except when the child is asleep, and exaggerated by slight causes.

A limited amount of crying is useful exercise for a baby, and should not distress his mother unduly. Moreover, crying may be merely the expression of a wish to be taken up, to be played with, carried about or otherwise amused, to be given a pacifier, or to be indulged in other bad habits. If not indulged in these ways he may cry from temper. The cry of temper is loud and violent, accompanied by vigorous kicking or by holding the body rigid. Proper treatment of the baby may prevent many months of discomfort, and spare him the formation of his first bad habit. All other possible causes for crying should be eliminated. If the child continues to cry when he is warm and dry and comfortable, "It should simply be allowed to cry it out. This often requires an hour and in extreme cases two or three hours. A second struggle will seldom last more than ten or fifteen minutes and a third will rarely be necessary" (Holt). Gas may form in the child's stomach during prolonged crying. It is consequently permissible to take him up after 15 minutes, and hold him erect; he generally expels gas at once, and immediately experiences relief. As soon as he is relieved, he should go back to his crib.

EXERCISE.--Exercise is essential to the development of the body, but during the first few weeks warmth and quiet are so important that a baby should not be disturbed except for necessary care. His position, however, should be changed occasionally; if he lies on the same side constantly the soft bones of the head may become misshapen from pressure. As the baby grows older he needs more exercise, and he may be given an opportunity for it by removing his outer clothing and placing him on a bed in a warm room for a short time each day. Unnecessary handling is not good for a baby at any age.

After he becomes more active, he may play on a mattress or thick blanket placed on the floor. The blanket should be covered with a washable pad or rubber cloth and clean sheet, and the whole should be surrounded by a fence at least two feet high. In such an enclosure a baby may safely be left to play if protected from draughts and cold. Elevated pens that can be folded when not in use are more convenient but more expensive than the home-made arrangement. As soon as a child begins to run about he takes ample exercise, and he may even need to be guarded from too great fatigue, especially toward bedtime. Games and play should be adapted to the age of the child and sufficiently varied to exercise all portions of the body; but they should not be too violent nor too prolonged. Some supervision of children's play is necessary, but they should be given as much freedom as possible and allowed to develop their own initiative.

PLAY AND TOYS.--The desire for play does not develop until a child is about six months old. At this age toys that can be washed, such as those of hard or soft rubber, should be selected. A baby instinctively carries everything to his mouth,--first his thumb, then playthings, and later whatever he may find, no matter how unsuitable. For his safety and protection this habit should be overcome as soon as possible, and he must learn to put nothing in his mouth except food and drink. Relatives are nearly always tempted to give too many and too fragile toys; they merely teach a child to be destructive and constantly to expect something new. Toys are the first possessions of which a child is conscious, and through them many desirable qualities may be developed: neatness and order, gentleness and a feeling of protection toward the helpless doll or Teddy bear, and unselfishness in sharing special treasures with playmates. Later the child may be given pets and made responsible for their care; but animals should not be subjected to unintentional cruelties from small children.

EXERCISES

1. What two factors are chiefly responsible for the deaths of babies under a year old? What other factors contribute? In your city or town what is the number of deaths per 1000 births of babies under one year old?

2. Why is birth registration important to an individual? to a community? Is it required by law in your city?

3. What is the average weight of babies at birth? Describe the rate at which they should gain.

4. At what age may a normal child be expected to sit erect? to stand? to walk? to speak? When should his first teeth appear? his permanent teeth?

5. Describe normal bowel movements of a baby.

6. How should a young baby be dressed?

7. Describe a baby's bath and toilet.

8. Describe the surroundings that are suitable for a baby.

9. What is the best food for a healthy baby? Why?

10. Describe in detail a good daily program for a healthy baby four months old.

11. What habits are desirable for a baby to form, and how may he be trained so that he will form them?

12. Name all the indications that would tell you when a baby was not thriving, and in each case tell what you would do about it.

FOR FURTHER READING

The Care and Feeding of Children--Holt.

The Care and Feeding of the Baby--Truby King.

The Baby's First Two Years--R. M. Smith.

The Care and Feeding of Children--J. L. Morse.

Preventive Medicine and Hygiene--Rosenau, Section III, Chapter II.

Pamphlets:

Prenatal Care, Mrs. Max West.

Infant Care, Mrs. Max West.

Child Care, Mrs. Max West. Published by the Children's Bureau, United States Department of Labor, Washington, D. C. (Free on request.)

The Care of the Baby--Supplement No. 10 to the Public Health
Reports, 1913, Government Printing Office, Washington, D. C.

Your Baby: How to Keep It Well--New York State Department of
Health, Albany.

Publications of the American Association for the Study and Prevention
of Infant Mortality--1211 Cathedral Street, Baltimore, Md. (Free on
request.)

Publications of the National Committee for the Prevention of
Blindness--130 East 22d Street, New York City. (Free on request.)

FOOTNOTES:

[1] An area including about two-thirds of the population of the United
States.

CHAPTER IV

INDICATIONS OF SICKNESS

By indications of sickness we mean all evidences of deviation from a normal physical condition. They may be apparent only to the person in whom they occur, or to a second person only, or to both. These deviations, commonly called the symptoms of sickness, are always important to notice, whether the conditions they indicate are serious or not.

Early symptoms of sickness are often slight; hence they easily pass unnoticed. Yet a slight trouble, easily checked in its early stages, may, if neglected, grow into a serious or even fatal disorder: just as a burning match, which anyone could extinguish instantly, may kindle a fire beyond the power of an entire city to control.

It is important, then, to notice even slight symptoms of sickness, first, in order to determine the nature of the trouble, and second, in order to institute treatment as early as possible. It is, however, hardly less important to observe symptoms accurately during the entire course of an illness. A patient's progress can be determined only by careful comparison between present and past conditions.

Many symptoms can be detected only by methods requiring scientific apparatus as well as the knowledge and skill of a physician, but very pronounced symptoms are generally evident to anyone. The neighbors do not need to be told when a person has advanced tuberculosis; neither is an expert required to see that something ails a man with a broken leg. Furthermore less pronounced symptoms may often be clearly seen by any observant person, even by those not specially trained. Accordingly it is important for every woman who has charge of others, sick or well, to form the habit of noticing unusual appearances of any kind. This habit is one that most people must take pains to acquire, because people generally see only the things that their own experience in life has taught them to see. An added difficulty is the fact that when illness begins it is not a trained observer, but the untrained sufferer or untrained member of his family who decides whether to send for the doctor and thus to set in motion the machinery for treatment and cure.

All the training and experience of a physician are required in order to decide what symptoms indicate, and to prescribe proper remedies. Diagnosis, or the process of determining the nature of illness from the symptoms observed, is often exceedingly difficult; it must take into consideration not one symptom only but the presence or absence of a number of symptoms. Untrained persons who attempt to make diagnoses are frequently led astray by the fact that actual causes of trouble may be situated far from the places where symptoms are felt or observed. For instance, the real cause of headache may lie in a region far removed from the head; and so-called heart-burn, which is caused by disordered digestion, has nothing to do with the heart. Again, an early symptom of tuberculosis of the hip joint is pain under the knee; a mother is clearly not doing the best thing when she assumes that any pain in a joint means rheumatism, and therefore doses her suffering child with the medicine that "helped" his rheumatic grandfather. No untrained person is equipped to make a diagnosis, and still less to prescribe medicine or treatment.

Symptoms, like all other forms of discomfort, tend to trouble a patient in proportion to the amount of attention that he gives them. Hence, in order to avoid calling his attention to them unnecessarily they should be observed so far as possible without his knowledge; when it is unavoidable for him to realize what is going on, observation should be made a matter of routine, so that his interest may not be especially excited. For instance, everyone who has seen the routine medical inspection of school children realizes how little attention the children themselves give to the process, apparently regarding it merely as one of the many inexplicable proceedings of grown people. On the other hand, children who know their symptoms are over-anxiously watched soon learn to watch themselves and to exaggerate every little ache and pain.

Symptoms may be divided into two classes: first, objective symptoms, or those that can be noted by an observer, like cough, pulse rate, or color of the skin; and second, the subjective symptoms, which are apparent only to the person affected, like pain and fatigue. The success of any woman who cares for the sick depends to a large

extent upon her quickness and accuracy in noticing and reporting
these symptoms and their variations. It should be remembered that
pronounced symptoms are not the only ones of importance: even slight
symptoms that continue over an appreciable length of time may be of
very great importance. A brief description of some important symptoms
follows, in order to help persons without technical training to describe
the symptoms as well as to observe them.

OBJECTIVE SYMPTOMS

TEMPERATURE.--Bodily heat is produced by slow burning of food
materials, which goes on for the most part in actively working muscles
and glands. Heat thus generated is distributed by the blood to all parts
of the body, but the surface of the body is generally cooler than the
interior. In health the body temperature varies only a few degrees, no
matter how much the temperature of its surroundings varies;
consequently a temperature is abnormal if it is higher or lower than the
usual temperature of a healthy person.

The temperature is taken by means of a clinical thermometer placed
either in the mouth, the rectum, or the armpit (axilla).

[Illustration: FIG. 10.--CLINICAL THERMOMETER.]

To take the mouth temperature, first wash the thermometer, using cold
water and absorbent cotton or clean soft cloth. Next shake it until the
mercury thread registers 96° or below. It is well before purchasing a
thermometer to see whether it can be shaken down easily. Next place
the thermometer in the patient's mouth, with its bulb under his tongue;
he must then keep his lips closed until it is removed. Leave the
thermometer in his mouth for two minutes. Then remove the
thermometer, read the temperature and record the result. Clean the
thermometer at once, using first cold water and soap, and then
alcohol, 70%.

The mouth temperature of a healthy person is about 98.6° F. This
statement holds true if the person has been sitting with his mouth shut
for a little while before his temperature is taken; but a hot bath,
breathing through the mouth, eating or drinking, and so forth may

cause marked temporary changes.

The temperature in the rectum generally varies less than the temperature in the mouth unless it is taken when the rectum contains fecal matter. The temperature should be taken by rectum in babies and young children, restless, drowsy, or delirious patients, patients who cannot be trusted to keep the thermometer under the tongue, mouth breathers, and in any patients who have difficulty in keeping the mouth shut. The temperature is normally about half a degree higher in the rectum than in the mouth.

In order to take a temperature by rectum, adults generally find it more convenient to lie on the side and prefer, if they are able, to insert and hold the thermometer themselves; but the attendant should be certain that they can do so without breaking the thermometer. Rectal thermometers should be lubricated with oil or vaseline before using; they should be inserted about two inches, left in three minutes, and cleansed in the same way as the mouth thermometer. A thermometer used to take rectal temperatures should never be used in the mouth.

In taking the temperature of a baby place him on his back, hold him firmly with his legs elevated, and carefully insert the bulb of the thermometer, well oiled, for about one inch. Keep the child quiet, and hold the thermometer in place three minutes. Great importance should not be attached to a slight fever of short duration. The temperature of a child is much more easily affected by slight causes than that of an adult, and rectal temperatures between 97.5° and 100.5° should not cause anxiety unless continued.

Temperatures taken in the axilla are less accurate than those taken by mouth or rectum. Consequently the method is less often used. The axilla should first be wiped; then the thermometer should be inserted and held for 5 minutes by pressing the arm tightly against the chest wall. The temperature in the axilla is normally about half a degree lower than in the mouth.

The temperature varies somewhat according to the time of day. It is not unusual for the mouth temperature of persons who are entirely healthy to be as low as 97° in the early morning, or as high as 99° in the late afternoon, and probably most people's temperatures vary as much as a degree during the twenty-four hours. Even greater variations that are not long continued have little if any significance in people who feel well.

Decided variations either above or below normal are highly important symptoms. A temperature below 98° is called subnormal, and one above 99.5° is called fever. The number of degrees of fever does not necessarily bear a direct relation to the severity of an illness. Thus, it does not follow that one person is twice as sick as another, because his temperature is twice as many degrees above normal. All symptoms, including variations in temperature, must be considered in connection with one another, and it is generally impossible to state the significance of any one symptom taken by itself.

The temperature should be taken once or twice a day as a matter of routine in almost every form of illness, and oftener when the patient's condition requires it. Also it should be taken as a matter of routine whenever there is indication of beginning sickness; especially when there is headache, pain, sore throat, coated tongue, cough or cold, chill, vomiting, diarrhoea, or rash. It is not a good plan to take one's own temperature oftener than necessary, or indeed anyone's; certainly not a baby's, since frequent use of the thermometer may irritate the rectum.

PULSE.--Each time the heart beats, blood is forced out from the heart into the arteries, thus causing an expansion of the arterial walls. This expansion, called the pulse, can be felt in some places where arteries lie close to the surface of the body. The character of the pulse beat and its rate, or the number of times the beat occurs each minute, give information about the heart and blood vessels; taken together they are perhaps more important than any other one symptom.

[Illustration: FIG. 11.--TAKING THE PULSE AT THE WRIST. NOTE THE POSITION OF ARM. (*From "Elementary Nursing Procedures," California State Board of Health.*)]

The pulse rate varies much more than the temperature. It differs in different individuals and at different ages, and it often shows great temporary changes, especially during exercise or eating, or as a result of excitement, fear, or other emotion. Definite statements in regard to normal pulse rates are hard to make, because different individuals though in perfect health show marked variations; we generally say, however, that the pulse rate of a normal man at rest is about 72 a minute, and that of a normal woman is about 80 a minute. At birth the pulse is quickest; it may then be from 124 to 144. From the 6th to the 12th month it may be from 105 to 115 a minute, and from 90 to 105 between the 2d and 6th years. About the time of puberty it reaches the adult rate, and during old age it may be decidedly slower than the adult rate.

What we chiefly want to know about the pulse is

1. Its rate, or number of beats per minute,

2. Its force,--whether weak or strong,

3. Its rhythm,--whether regular or irregular.

Much practice is necessary before the pulse rate can be counted with any degree of accuracy, and wide experience with both normal and abnormal pulses is required in order to judge its strength, rhythm, or other characteristics.

The pulse may be felt most conveniently on the thumb side of the front of the wrist. The pulse should be counted while the patient is lying down, and the watch used must have a second hand. To count the pulse, one should place two or three fingers (not the thumb) on the patient's wrist, and after the pulse has been felt distinctly for a few beats, the exact time by the second hand of the watch should be noticed and the counting begun immediately. It is generally best to count for half a minute, multiply the result by two to get the rate for a whole minute, and then to repeat for another half minute. The two results should agree within two beats, if the patient is quiet. A greater variation than two beats may mean that the pulse rate is varying, but when it is counted by inexperienced persons the apparent difference is generally the result of inaccurate counting, and it may be necessary to count two or three times more. The force of the pulse varies also in different individuals; it is, however, important to notice when it grows stronger or weaker in the same person. Normally the pulse-beat is regular like the ticking of a clock; it is called irregular if a few rapid or slow beats are followed by others of a different rate. During sickness the pulse should be counted whenever the temperature is taken, or oftener; and the result should be written down at once. The pulse of a sick person often shows changes both in rate and character; these changes are generally important and should be noticed.

RESPIRATION.--Variations in the rate and character of respiration or breathing should be noticed. The normal rate of respiration for an adult at rest is 16 to 20 each minute, but it may be much faster, especially during muscular exercise. In babies the rate is about 30 to 35 a minute, and 20 to 25 in little children. The respirations, especially of babies, can best be counted during sleep by placing the hand lightly on the chest or abdomen. Since the respiration rate is partly under a person's control, it is almost sure to alter if the patient knows it is being counted; hence when the patient is awake it is better to keep one's fingers on his wrist, to place his hand upon his chest, and then to count the rise and fall of the chest while apparently counting the pulse. Sometimes it is possible to count the respirations merely by watching the rise and fall of the nightgown or bed clothes. The respiration is usually counted for a full minute. A watch with a second hand must be used, and the result should be recorded immediately.

In certain forms of sickness breathing may become rapid, especially if the lungs or air passages are affected. In addition to the rate anything unusual about the breathing should be noticed whether it seems difficult or painful; if noisy, whether the sound is like snoring, or wheezing, or sighing, and so on.

GENERAL APPEARANCE.--Any unusual expression of the face should be noted; whether it is drawn, pinched, anxious, excited, or dull and stupid; and also, whether the face is thin, swollen, or puffy under the eyes. The condition and appearance of the skin are significant: the skin may be dry, moist and clammy, hot or cold; its color, and the color of the face especially, may be flushed or pale or slightly yellow or blue. A bluish tinge about the nose, tips of the fingers, or the feet should be specially noticed. Reddened or discolored areas on any part of the body may be important, and also eruptions, rashes, swellings, or sores. It should be noticed whether the abdomen is normal or whether it is distended and hard.

Strength or weakness is indicated to some extent by the way the patient moves, and by his ability to walk, stand, sit, hold up his head, feed himself, or turn in bed without assistance. The position he habitually takes is sometimes significant; in heart affections, for instance, he may be unable to lie down, in pleurisy he ordinarily lies on the affected side, and during abdominal pain he generally draws the knees up.

SPECIAL SENSES.--The special senses are frequently disturbed in sickness. The eyes may be blood-shot; the patient may be over-sensitive to light, or see spots floating before the eyes, or he may be unable to see at all. The pupils of the eyes may be unusually large or small, or one may be large while the other is small. Swelling, redness, or discharge from the eyes should be noticed. Hearing and touch and smell may be impaired; or they may be abnormally acute, and cause real suffering. Taste may be impaired, especially when the nose is affected or when the mouth is not clean. Discharge from the nose or ears should be reported. Not only discharge, but also trouble of any kind, such as pain, tenderness, or swelling, is important if situated in or near the ears.

THE VOICE is often much altered in sickness. It may be weak, hoarse, or whispered. Speech may be clear or thick, or the ability to speak may be entirely lost; in extreme weakness speaking is generally difficult, and may be impossible. Moaning, groaning, and other unusual sounds should be noted. A loud, sharp cry at night with or without waking, if a repeated occurrence, may be an early symptom of some diseases of children.

THE TONGUE in health is red and moist; when extended it is somewhat pointed and can be held steadily. In sickness it may be cracked, dry and parched, or if the patient is not properly cared for, it may be covered with white, yellow, or brown coating; in many exhausting illnesses it is flabby and trembling. In scarlet fever the tongue is often a vivid red color, and is then called strawberry tongue.

The odor of the breath may be foul from decay or neglect of the teeth, from indigestion, constipation, nasal catarrh, or special diseases.

THE THROAT and tonsils are sometimes red and swollen as in simple sore throat; or they may be covered by white patches.

THE GUMS may be swollen, tender, or bleeding. A collection of sticky brownish material may appear on the teeth and gums of neglected patients.

COUGH when present may be: dry, or accompanied by expectoration; painful, frequent, loud, or whooping; and worse by day or by night. The sputum may be yellow, white, gray, rusty, blood-streaked, dark, or frothy. The amount of sputum should be noticed as well as its appearance.

APPETITE or absence of appetite should be noted, and also the amount of food actually eaten by a patient; the amount eaten is frequently not the same as the amount carried to him on a tray.

If VOMITING occurs, the color, consistency, amount, and general appearance of the vomitus should be noted; if its appearance is unusual the vomitus should be saved for the doctor's inspection.

EXCRETIONS.--The number of bowel movements is important, and also their character. The consistency of the feces may be hard, soft or fluid; their color may be any shade of brown, yellow or green, from black to clay color. They should be saved for the doctor to see if appearance or odor is unusual.

THE URINE in health is clear, amber colored, and slightly acid. From 30 to 50 ounces should be excreted in 24 hours; the amount varies, however, especially according to the amount of fluid taken. It is important to notice whether the urine is scanty or greatly increased in amount, dark or pale, clear or cloudy, and whether sediment is deposited after standing. It is essential that urine should be voided in sufficient amount; the necessity for watching its quantity is frequently overlooked in the home care of the sick. Frequency of urination should also be noted. Inability to urinate, particularly where the urine has previously been scanty, is serious if continued; it should be reported to the doctor without delay. Inability to control the bladder and bowels are also symptoms to be reported.

LOSS OF WEIGHT is significant in both adults and children, and failure of babies and children to gain in weight is a danger signal.

SLEEP.--The number of hours a patient sleeps should be noticed and recorded as accurately as possible. The word of the patient on this subject is not sufficient evidence. Character of sleep should also be noted, whether it is quiet or restless, and whether the patient sleeps lightly or is difficult to arouse.

MENTAL CONDITIONS.--It is important to watch carefully the mental condition of a patient; whether, for example, he is normal, or depressed, irritable, restless, apathetic, dull, excited, wandering, delirious, or unconscious. Hasty judgment of mental conditions should be avoided, but close attention to them is necessary.

SUBJECTIVE SYMPTOMS

PAIN is the most important subjective symptom and should never be disregarded. Bodily pain does not occur in persons who are in all regards physically and mentally well; hence pain is a sign that something, small or great, is out of order.

"Of all symptoms pain is the one which interests patients the most. We here emphasize the truth, too little understood, that pain is an unpleasant sensation, nothing more, and is *never* imagined. Imagination may be its cause, but the pain thus produced hurts just as truly as pain produced by a real disease. Pain is only a phenomenon of consciousness; it is always real, even that felt in a dream. If the patient is too unconscious to feel it, there simply is no pain, no matter how badly the person's body is injured." (Emerson: Essentials of Medicine, p. 356.)

One should remember that no possible method exists to measure the intensity of pain exactly, or to describe its quality accurately. Therefore in describing pain, it is best to use the patient's own language. Four points should especially be observed, (1) its location; (2) its character, which may be dull or sharp, stabbing, throbbing or continuous, slight or severe; (3) the time at which it is worst; certain diseases, for instance, are characterized by more severe pain at night; (4) it should be noticed whether the pain is relieved or increased by change of position, eating or drinking, heat or cold, or the like. Pain may be felt in a part far from the place where the trouble really lies; thus a dislocated shoulder causes pain in the elbow.

Pain is always a danger signal, although the significance is not always so great as the sufferer thinks. The more attention a patient gives to his pain, the more severe it always becomes, therefore his attention should not be called to it unnecessarily. A good observer, however, can get much information by noticing the patient's expression, position, motions, etc., without constantly asking him how he feels. Although many persons overestimate pain, others persistently disregard it, either because they are unwilling to take the necessary measures to remedy it, or because they wish to appear heroic. Both courses of action are mistaken; everyone should realize the folly and danger of bearing pain if it is possible to remove the cause.

Nausea, fatigue and malaise are other subjective symptoms; malaise is the name given to a general feeling of physical discomfort not restricted to any one part of the body. All three are abnormal when there is not apparent or sufficient cause.

RECORDS.--An accurate record should be kept of the patient's symptoms, medicine, diet, treatment, etc., so that the doctor may have a continuous record, and so that another person taking charge temporarily may know just what has been done for the patient. The record must be written; otherwise details cannot be remembered exactly. It should be as simple and concise as possible; it is the place for facts, not for opinions, and if inaccurate it is worse than none. It is better not to keep the record in the patient's room, for the patient should not see his own record, nor hear its contents discussed. The doctor usually writes his orders on the record sheet itself, or on a separate sheet to be attached to the record for reference. Blank record forms can be purchased, but a form that is made at home is entirely satisfactory. An example of a daily record sheet follows.

RECORD

```
------+-----------+----+-----+-----+---------------+----+-----+------- Date | Hour
|Tem.|Pulse|Resp.| Diet and |B.M.|Urine|Remarks | | | | | medicine | | |
------+-----------+----+-----+-----+---------------+----+-----+------- 1916 | | | | | |
| | Jan. 1|4 p.m. |100°| 76 | 24 |Medicine | | | |5 p.m. | | | | | 1 |oz. | | | | | |
| |vii | |6 p.m. | | | |Supper: | | | | | | | | Baked potato, | | | | | | | | toast, fruit,
| | | | | | | | tea. | | | |8 p.m. | | | |Medicine | | |Sponge | | | | | | |bath. |9:30
p.m. | | | | | | |Asleep. Jan. 2|3 a.m. | | | | | |oz. | | | | | | | |ix | |8 a.m. |99° |
74 | 22 |Medicine | | |Patient | | | | | | | |slept | | | | | | | |most | | | | | | | |of
the | | | | | | | |night. |8:30 a.m. | | | |Breakfast: | | | | | | | | Cereal, orange,|
| | | | | | | | toast, coffee. | | | |9:30 a.m. | | | |Bath. | | | |11:30 a.m.| | | | | |
|Sat up | | | | | | | |1 hour.
------+-----------+----+-----+-----+---------------+----+-----+-------
```

TUBERCULOSIS, CANCER, AND MENTAL ILLNESS.--As we have
seen, early symptoms of sickness are always important; yet it seems
worth while to mention particularly the early symptoms of tuberculosis,
cancer, and mental disorders, because each of these diseases, though
curable in many cases when taken in the early stages, is serious and
often fatal if neglected. Certain facts relating to their cause and
prevention should be known to everyone. Tuberculosis, long our
greatest cause of death, is gradually growing less; but cancer and
mental disease are now on the increase.

TUBERCULOSIS.--Every year tuberculosis causes the death of about
150,000 people in the United States. It is caused by the bacillus
tuberculosis, a germ which may attack any tissue of the body, although
it most frequently affects the lungs of grown people, and the bones and
glands of children. The disease is not inherited, but susceptibility to it
appears to be; it is readily communicated from person to person. The
germ of tuberculosis is so widely distributed that probably few persons
over 30 years of age have not been infected with it at some time,
although the infection may have been too slight to be noticed. Indeed,
most people have probably been infected many times, though without
serious results.

Tuberculosis is spread chiefly in two ways: (1) through any bodily
discharges from infected persons, especially through the nose and

mouth discharges; (2) through milk from infected cows. The ways by which the disease is spread indicate methods of prevention. Milk, especially for children, should either be pasteurized or should come from cows that have been tested and proved to be free from the disease. Other methods of prevention include avoiding any and all bodily discharges of infected persons, and increasing bodily resistance as far as possible. Good food, sufficient rest and fresh air are not only important preventives, but also the most efficacious means of cure. Persons who suffer from insufficient food, exposure, bad housing, long hours, and bad conditions of work are especially susceptible to tuberculosis, and thus it is rightly called a disease of poverty.

Early symptoms of tuberculosis include cough, hoarseness, loss of appetite, pain in the side, loss of weight, getting tired easily, feeling run down, rise in temperature in the afternoon, night sweats, expectoration, and spitting blood. No one, nor even several, of these symptoms necessarily indicates the presence of tuberculosis; on the other hand, even the cough is not necessarily present when tuberculosis actually exists. When one or more of these symptoms appears and continues, a thorough examination should be made by a doctor; examination can do no harm, certainly, if tuberculosis is not found, and if it is, immediate treatment is of the greatest importance. No known drug or medicine is a cure for tuberculosis. Successful treatment depends on taking the disease in time and in following the doctor's advice unremittingly.

CANCER.--The cause of cancer is not known. All the evidence, however, goes to show that it is neither communicable nor hereditary. Cancer may occur on the skin, stomach, or other organs; in women it most commonly occurs in the breast or uterus (womb). In both sexes it occurs most frequently after 40 years of age. No known medicine will cure cancer; salves and ointments have no effect. Radium and *x*-ray should not be relied upon if the cancer can be removed by operation. Safety consists in removing the growth entirely, and complete removal is possible only in the early stages.

Early diagnosis is consequently of the greatest possible importance, and an examination can do no harm in any case. Warts and moles on the skin may develop into cancer, and should be removed if they show signs of irritation. Loss of appetite and weight, any disturbance of the stomach or intestines, and sores that refuse to heal should lead a person to consult a physician; the same is true of any lump in the breast, and of irregular or persistent bleeding from the uterus in women over forty. The fact that pain is not present in cancer until the late stages leads many persons to neglect the trouble until it is too far advanced for operation. Time is all-important; hope depends on operation in the early stages when there is a very great probability of permanent cure.

MENTAL ILLNESS.--Insanity, like cancer, is increasing. Like both cancer and tuberculosis, hope lies in prevention and early treatment; and like them both, in its early symptoms it is too often unrecognized or neglected.

Many people are surprised to learn that known, avoidable causes are responsible for the condition of about 50% of the insane patients now under treatment. Chief among these known causes is a communicable germ disease called syphilis, to which is due the disease called paresis, or "softening of the brain." About 25% of patients admitted to hospitals for the insane are there from the effects of habitual use of alcohol, even in "moderate" quantities. Other cases of insanity result from diseases of the heart, arteries, and kidneys, and still others have been traced to the poisons of tuberculosis, typhoid, diphtheria, and other communicable diseases. Prevention of insanity caused by these diseases depends upon prevention or complete cure of the diseases themselves.

Still other causes of insanity are known. Hereditary nervous weakness may predispose to insanity, and for such persons, those whose nervous resistance is naturally not very great, the stress of living may prove too much. Mental breakdowns are rarely caused by overwork unless accompanied by worry or bad hygienic conditions, but they result not infrequently from bad mental habits.

"The average person, little realizes the danger of brooding over slights, injuries, disappointments, or misfortunes, or of an unnatural attitude towards his fellowmen, shown by unusual sensitiveness or marked suspicion. Yet all these unwholesome and painful trains of thought, may if persisted in and unrelieved by healthy interests and activities, tend towards insanity. Wholesome work relieved by periods of rest and simple pleasures and an interest in the affairs of others, are important preventives of unwholesome ways of thinking. We should train ourselves not to brood, but to honestly face personal difficulties."--(Why Should Anyone Go Insane?, by Folks and Ellwood.)

Prevention of insanity consequently depends chiefly upon avoiding alcohol and communicable diseases, especially syphilis; upon good hygiene, self-control, and avoidance of bad mental habits; and upon adopting a program of living and working that will not overtax one's nervous strength. Sleeplessness, unusual nervous fatigue following slight exertion, and diminished power to control the emotions, are among the danger signals. And when a person becomes unusually depressed or morose, excited or irritable, suspicious, unreasonable, or "queer," it is probable that expert medical advice should be obtained as quickly as possible.

EXERCISES

1. What is a symptom? Why are early symptoms especially important?

2. Distinguish between objective and subjective symptoms.

3. Tell all you can about normal and abnormal variations in the body temperature. What symptoms would lead you to take a person's temperature?

4. Describe the method of taking temperatures.

5. How should you cleanse a clinical thermometer? What are the dangers of neglecting to cleanse it properly?

6. Describe both normal and abnormal pulse and respiration.

7. Discuss the significance and importance of pain.

8. Describe early symptoms of tuberculosis, cancer, and mental illness. What is the first step to be taken when any one of these

symptoms appears?

9. What symptoms of all those mentioned in this chapter did you notice in the last sick person with whom you had anything to do?

10. What are the essentials of a good daily record? The following is an account that a mother gave of the first twenty-four hours of a child's illness. Make a chart for the patient, and include in it all the information the mother gave. Which do you consider more useful, your chart or the narrative?

"Yesterday, October 10th, Johnny came home from school about half past three, and said he was too cold to play outdoors. He lay down and slept till about five, when he vomited a large amount of undigested food. I took his temperature and found that it was 103.8°, pulse 126, and respiration 28. At 10 that night his temperature was 102.5°, pulse 116, and respiration the same as before. The next morning at 8 he had a temperature of 100.6°, pulse 114, respiration 24. At noon his temperature was 101°, pulse 118, respiration 24; and at 4 o'clock his temperature was 100.6°, pulse 122, respiration 22. The doctor came at 6 o'clock yesterday afternoon; according to his orders I put Johnny to bed, gave him half a tablespoonful of castor oil at 6.30, and a special gargle. His throat was red and sore and he seemed to feel very miserable. The doctor took a culture from the child's throat. At 8.15 and again at 8.50 he had fluid bowel movements. At 9.30 he had a glass of milk, after which he slept until 6 a.m. when his bowels moved again and urine was passed. He passed eight ounces of urine at noon and four ounces at 3.30. He drank a glass of water at 6 this morning, and at 6.30 I gave him a cup of hot broth. At 8 he had a glass of milk, but at 10 he refused everything but a glass of water. At 1.30 he had a large dish of ice cream. He had a cool sponge bath last night at 9, and a cleansing bath this morning at 8.45. This morning his throat was still sore but not so red, and I saw that he gargled every half hour when he was awake. This afternoon he seems brighter and asked for his harmonica, so his throat is probably more comfortable."

FOR FURTHER READING

Essentials of Medicine--Emerson, Chapters XVI, XVII.

The Human Mechanism--Hough and Sedgwick, Chapter XII.

Notes on Nursing--Florence Nightingale, Pages 105-136.

Why Worry?--Walton.

Those Nerves--Walton.

Tuberculosis: Its Cause, Cure, and Prevention--Otis.

Publications of the National Association for the Study and Prevention of Tuberculosis--105 East 22d Street, New York City. (Pamphlets free on request.)

Publications of the National Committee for Mental Hygiene--50 Union Square, New York City. (Pamphlets free on request.)

Publications of the Mental Hygiene Committee of the State Charities Aid Association--105 East 22d Street, New York City. (Pamphlets free on request.)

Publications of The American Society for the Control of Cancer--25 West 45th Street, New York City. (Pamphlets free on request.)

CHAPTER V

EQUIPMENT AND CARE OF THE SICK ROOM

Adequate care of the sick consists to a large extent in rendering their physical and mental surroundings as favorable as possible. Obviously, a sick person, since his strength is already depleted, needs not only to have his resistance increased in all possible ways, but also to have all his remaining strength conserved by eliminating every unnecessary tax upon it. In sickness even slight fatigue, chill, or nervous strain, insufficient ventilation, or improper feeding, may become factors of immense importance. Nothing is trivial if it affects the welfare and comfort of a patient.

Even when perfect provision for the care of the sick is out of the question, every effort should be made to insure as satisfactory arrangements as possible. Ideal conditions are seldom found except in buildings originally planned for the sick; yet in many houses a few simple changes will produce excellent results. Of course, it is not necessary in every case to adopt all the following suggestions. Common sense must be the guide. For instance, in illness that is slight and likely to be of short duration, a patient may be more distressed than benefited by radical changes in his surroundings. Except when certain essentials are concerned, great consideration should be given to a patient's preferences; yet on the other hand it is not reasonable to make an entire family miserable in order to gratify some slight whim.

CHOICE OF A SICK ROOM.--A south or east exposure is generally best for a sick room. A south room may be undesirable in very hot weather, but sunshine during a part of the day is essential. The room should be quiet, near the bath room, and well removed from odors from the kitchen. It should be situated so that good ventilation is possible. It is desirable though not necessary for it to have more than one window; in summer the windows must be thoroughly screened. It should be possible to open the window without exposing the patient to a direct current of air, and to open the door without placing him in full view of all who pass through the hall.

It is essential for the patient to have a room to himself. Unless he needs care or help or watching at night, not even the person caring for him should sleep in the room. Neither should the rest of the family keep their possessions in the sick room. Closets opening into the room, bureaus, and chiffoniers should be emptied of the belongings of other members of the family, to prevent people from tiptoeing into the sick room at all hours to remove garments. The sick room should for the time belong exclusively to the patient, and resulting inconvenience should be borne by well members of the family.

Every possible precaution should be taken to exclude from a sick room unnecessary noises of all kinds; flapping curtains, squeaky doors and rocking chairs, heels without rubber, creaking corsets, noisy petticoats, ticking clocks, refractory bureau drawers, and rustling newspapers are among the everyday sounds that irritate the nerves of sick and well alike. Ordinary out-of-door noises do not usually disturb the sick, except when the country patient is brought to the city, or the reverse; but nearby and generally avoidable noise is the kind that distracts and harasses nervous patients.

Whispering is an annoying sound and should not be allowed, either in the patient's room or just outside the door. Whatever the subject of conversation may be, the patient thinks that he is under discussion. Anything undesirable for him to hear should be settled well out of his hearing, and in speaking to him there is no possible objection to an ordinary well modulated voice.

Usually a person's own room is more restful and less disturbing than a strange place, but if it serves as a work room as well as a bed room, it may easily be the worst place during sickness. The sight of a desk piled high with papers or a basket overflowing with accumulations of family mending may actually delay recovery; even the room itself may constantly suggest work, and work necessarily left undone. The essential thing to remember is that mental rest is no less important than physical, and every effort should be made to secure them both.

FURNISHING.--Superfluous articles add to the care of a sick room, and in consequence they should be removed at the outset. All the furnishings that remain should be easy to clean, but it is not necessary for a sick room to look bare and desolate.

The woodwork as in any other room should have a hard finish, and angles and corners that harbor dust should be as few as possible. Hard wood floors without cracks are best from the point of view of cleanliness and convenience. A few light, washable rugs make the best floor covering, but very small rugs on highly polished floors slide easily and are decidedly dangerous. Carpets diminish noise, but are objectionable from every other point of view.

In furnishing houses people ought to realize more frequently than they do how greatly nervous fatigue may be increased by ill chosen wall coverings. Plain papers or tinted walls are best for bed rooms and the color should not be harsh or striking; soft gray, green, or buff is good. The design is no less important than the color; a design that on casual inspection appears quite harmless may become an instrument of torture to a person unable to escape from it for a single hour. Weak or nervous patients sometimes become quite exhausted from attempting to follow an intricate pattern, or from counting over and over a design that is frequently repeated on the wall. If the patient sees grotesque faces and figures in the design the paper is more objectionable still.

Necessary furniture includes the bed, which will be discussed in detail later, a small table to stand by the head of the bed, a dresser, two chairs, and a wall thermometer. If the patient is able to sit up three chairs are needed, of which one should be an armchair with a high back. No rocking chair should be allowed in the room unless the patient himself prefers to sit in one; no one else should be allowed to rock in the room, since the motion is almost always annoying to patients. Elaborate, carved, or upholstered furniture is unsuitable in a sick room, but if it must be used it should have washable covers.

Other desirable articles of furniture are a couch, screen, foot-stool and a second, larger table. In few cases, if any, is anything further really necessary, although patients frequently desire special articles to which there can be no objection.

Most ornaments add much work and little beauty, and have no place in a sick-room. No heavy unwashable curtains or hangings should be allowed, but simple washable curtains and clean white covers for the tables and dresser are desirable. Pictures, if suitable, give much pleasure, but must be used with discretion. It goes without saying that the subjects should be pleasant, but not everyone realizes that complicated subjects are undesirable and that pictures of people or things in motion should be avoided; patients are sometimes worried to see motion that is forever incomplete.

Flowers give great pleasure to the sick by adding color and variety and interest to their surroundings. They should be carefully tended and given fresh water daily. Fading flowers and forlorn plants should be removed from the sick room, and those having strong, heavy odors should not even be admitted. They do not need to be very many or very expensive; indeed, a potted plant or a few cut flowers are often more acceptable than the great masses of costly flowers that are daily brought to the private wards of hospitals.

VENTILATION.--A patient needs fresh air certainly as much as a well person, and probably even more. His room should be thoroughly ventilated night and day. A fireplace makes the problem easier, but in most cases an open window is the main dependence. It should be possible to open windows at the top as well as at the bottom, and the patient may be protected from a direct draught by a screen, or by a sheet stretched along the side of the bed and fastened at the head and foot by tying it around the posts.

Ventilating a room without subjecting the patient to draughts is not always easy. One method is to insert a board three or four inches high under the lower sash so that air is admitted between the two sashes. Another way to ventilate without causing a draught is to remove one or two panes of glass and tack cheese cloth over the opening; or to tack cheese cloth to the lower edge of the upper window casing and to the upper edge of the upper sash, after the sash has been lowered about a foot. Once or twice a day the room should be thoroughly aired by opening windows and doors until the air has been completely changed. The patient, including his head, must be well-covered during the process. An electric fan is useful in summer, but it should not be close enough to the bed for the patient to feel air blowing upon him.

HEATING.--Great care should be taken to maintain a suitable temperature in the sick-room, and for this purpose a thermometer in the room is a necessity. Between 65° and 68° is generally the best temperature, and hot water bags and extra covers may be given if the patient is chilly. During a bath or other treatment in which the patient is more or less exposed the temperature should be 70°. The temperature at night may be lower; how low will depend largely on the patient's condition and on what must be done for him during the night. Hot water, steam heat, or electricity is best for the sick room. Gas or oil stoves should never be used except in emergencies, and then for a short time only.

LIGHTING.--Sunlight is one of the most powerful disinfectants, and for this reason if for no other it is needed in every sick room. Sunless rooms, moreover, even if they were wholesome, are too depressing to a patient's spirits for use except perhaps in hot summer days. Ordinary well-regulated light is best in a sick room, and except in a few diseases, especially those in which the eyes are affected, it is undesirable to darken the room or to encourage in any way an appearance of gloom. The patient's eyes, however, should be protected from bright lights shining directly upon them; in this connection it is well to remember that lights and their reflections strike differently upon the eyes of a person lying down from the way in which they strike the eyes of persons sitting or standing, and a light that seems agreeable to the attendant may therefore be painful to the patient.

Almost all persons sleep best in dark rooms, and in most cases it is undesirable for a sick room to be lighted at night. The attendant, however, must be able to see what she is doing and generally needs a shaded candle, small night light, or electric flash. It should be possible to see the patient clearly in case of need, otherwise serious changes in his condition occurring in the night may pass unnoticed.

A reading lamp on the bedside table is desirable for patients allowed to read, but reading in bed even with a well-regulated light is fatiguing, and should not be continued for long uninterrupted periods. A pocket flash light is safer than matches and a candle for patients who wish to consult their watches in the night; indeed, matches in the hands of patients always involve risk. Some patients find twilight a time of great depression. In such a case it had best be shortened by drawing the shades early, turning on the lights, and remembering not to leave him alone.

CLEANING.--The sick-room should be kept thoroughly clean at all times, and the less dust stirred up in doing so the better. Dry sweeping or dusting should not be allowed. Ordinary brooms should be dampened or covered with damp cloths, and dust cloths should be dampened also; but dustless mops and dusters are still better. Vacuum cleaning is very desirable; the noise, which is its only disadvantage, is not a serious objection in most cases. The cleaning of rooms after a communicable disease will be considered later.

A sick room must be kept tidy as well as clean. The effect of order is quieting, but it should be maintained whether the effect upon the patient is apparent or not. Food and medicine should not be kept in the sick-room, and all used dishes, tumblers, soiled linen, etc., should be removed at once. Unnecessary articles should not be found in the room at any time; every necessary article should be kept in its place, and its place should be a good one.

Maintaining order in the room does not mean that patients should be made uncomfortable. All patients, especially old people, want certain possessions within reach, and their wishes should be considered in spite of the fact that the æsthetic effect is generally far from good. For instance, a perfectly smooth bed is undesirable if in order to make it smooth the patient must be tucked in so tightly that he is uncomfortable. And it would be a mistake to remove an old man's newspapers before he has read them, even if he persists in strewing them all over the floor.

THE ATTENDANT.--One person and one person only should carry the entire responsibility for the patient. She should plan for him as well as care for him, should see the doctor and take the doctor's orders. Confusion and innumerable mistakes result when several members of the family attempt to do the talking and directing.

The attendant should wear washable dresses with sleeves that can be rolled up, washable aprons, and shoes with rubber heels. All her clothing should be comfortable. She should be neat in appearance, scrupulously clean in person, and should keep her finger nails short and smooth. Jewelry, especially rings and chains that rattle, and finery of any sort are all out of place in a sick-room.

The attendant must learn that her own sleep, her diet, and her out-of-door exercise are essential to the patient's well-being hardly less than to her own. An amateur nurse often considers that going without food and sleep is a proof of her devotion. In a passion of self-sacrifice she neglects herself utterly for the first few days, and as a consequence is quite useless at a later period when her services may be most needed. An exhausted, sleepy nurse, trained or untrained, is wholly unfit to be trusted with medicines and doctor's orders, to note changes in the patient's condition, or to give him kindly attention. Efficiency and fatigue have never pulled together since the world began, and no one can do good work when suffering from lack of sleep and rest.

The person, then, who genuinely wishes to give her patient the best possible care should not make a martyr of herself. She should go out of doors daily; both fresh air and occasional absence from the patient are essential to her physical and mental well-being. Moreover, she will be showing her patient the greatest kindness in the long run if during her recreation time she thinks of him as little as possible. Indeed, she need not consider herself inhuman if she has a thoroughly good time.

On the other hand, a person who is responsible for the care of a patient must be made to realize that she and she only is ultimately responsible during the entire 24 hours of every day. Being responsible for a patient does not mean that she should be with him every minute, or do everything herself: it does mean that she should plan so effectively that everything necessary is done, either by herself or by another competent person. When she goes away for even half an hour, she should appoint someone else to be responsible in her place and to her when she comes back. She must consequently make very clear just what she wants done. If there is medicine, nourishment, or treatment to be given, she can easily make a list, with the time for each, and ask that each item be crossed off the list as soon as the work has been done. She should not forget to ask for the list when she returns.

What is really needed is a little executive ability. As Florence Nightingale said:

"It is impossible in a book to teach a person in charge of the sick how to *manage*, as it is to teach her how to nurse. Circumstances must vary with each different case. But it is possible to press upon her to think for herself. Now what does happen during my absence? I am obliged to be away on Tuesday. But fresh air, or punctuality is not less important to my patient on Tuesday than it was on Monday. Or: At 10 p.m. I am never with my patient; but quiet is of no less consequence to him at 10 than it was at 5 minutes to 10. Curious as it may seem, this very obvious consideration occurs comparatively to few, or, if it does occur, it is only to cause the devoted friend or nurse to be absent fewer hours, or even fewer minutes from her patient--not to arrange so as that no minute and no hour shall be for her patient without the essentials of her nursing."--(Notes on Nursing.)

It is exceedingly difficult to care for members of one's own family or to be cared for by them. Too much or too little is almost invariably expected by one person or the other, and where great affection is involved not only is the strain increased on both sides, but often harm results from too great unselfishness on either side or both. But sometimes the reverse is true, and then one should remember that normal behavior may be impossible for the sick. During weakness and pain, irritability and unreasonableness are as characteristic as other symptoms, and it is as foolish to demand a normal mental state from a sick person as it would be to demand a normal temperature. For a cheerful, reasonable, and unselfish patient--and there are surprisingly many--one should be devoutly thankful, but patience and pity should be given no less to those whose tortured nerves cause suffering to others as well as to themselves.

Every woman who cares for the sick should remember that she is the patient's chief if not his only link with the normal world, and that his plight is pitiful indeed if she is complaining or irritable or unwilling.

Anyone who cares for the sick should remember also that she is necessarily in a most intimate relation with the patient, and that such enforced intimacy calls for extra consideration on her part, and for the most scrupulous respect for confidential matters. It is inexcusable even for members of the patient's family to discuss with one another the patient's private concerns, or his queer or unreasonable or annoying ways. During sickness the skeletons in most people's mental closets walk forth, and anyone who misuses special opportunities to know intimate affairs can only be classed with eavesdroppers and village gossips.

EXERCISES

1. What are the essentials of a good sick room as to:

(*a*) Situation and exposure. (*b*) Lighting and heating. (*c*) Furnishing. (*d*) Ventilation.

2. How may a sick room be ventilated without exposing the patient to draughts?

3. How should the bed be placed in relation to doors, windows, and walls?

4. How should a sick room be cleaned?

5. What in general are the duties of the attendant?

6. Make a plan of your own bedroom, and show what changes, if any, would be desirable if it were to be used as a sick room.

FOR FURTHER READING

Notes on Nursing--Florence Nightingale, Pages 1-63, 84-105.

CHAPTER VI

BEDS AND BEDMAKING

The common saying that the best bed for an invalid is his own bed contains an element of truth. Taking from a patient his own accustomed bed, even when a better is substituted, sometimes disturbs him greatly and makes him feel that he is indeed very ill. Nevertheless, a suitable bed is essential to the proper care of a helpless person, and no patient should continue to use an unsuitable one, unless his illness is slight and also likely to be of very short duration.

Besides being comfortable, a bed suitable for the sick must be clean and easy to keep in a sanitary condition. The springs should be firm, and the mattress should be elastic and should give an even support without lumps and hollows. The bed covers should be clean, light, and warm; the pillows should be sufficient in number not only to make the head and shoulders comfortable, but also any other part of the body in need of support. Moreover, the bed should be so placed and of such a kind that the work of caring for the patient may be rendered as easy for the attendant as possible. In every household at least one bed suitable for a sick person should be available in case of need.

BEDSTEADS.--Beds of white enameled iron, brass, or brass and iron combined are most easily kept clean, and are the best in every way. The frame should be strong enough to stand firmly, yet not so heavy that it is hard to move. It should have as few angles as possible, and all its joints should be smooth and well finished. The springs should be made of wire stretched tightly on a metal frame that fits smoothly into the head and foot pieces. Large castors should be used; they may be removed from the foot if the bed moves too easily.

A bed to be used in sickness should have the following dimensions--length, 6 ft. 6 in., height 24 to 26 inches, width, 36 inches. If a bed is either too high or too low the labor of lifting and moving the patient is greatly increased. If the bed is too narrow the patient is insecure. If the bed is too wide, its center is difficult or impossible to reach without leaning or kneeling upon it; and if too short, it will prove uncomfortable for a tall person. A bed that is too low may be raised on four heavy boxes of the same height; or still better, upon heavy wooden blocks which any carpenter can easily make, and which are well worth a little trouble to obtain. In the top of each block a hollow should be made into which the leg of the bed will fit after the castor has been removed. A broad firm stool or a low chair may be provided for a patient who has difficulty in getting in and out of a high bed.

Beds with complicated attachments for moving patients are not recommended for family use. They are expensive, likely to get out of order, seldom needed, and generally unsatisfactory. In some surgical cases a bed with a firm, flat surface is necessary. Such a surface may be secured by placing between the mattress and springs two boards slightly separated, or one wide board with holes bored in it to afford ventilation.

Wooden beds are undesirable: they are difficult to keep clean, they readily absorb moisture and odors, they cannot well be disinfected, and their solid frames prevent a free circulation of air. Moreover, it is almost impossible to render fit for use again a wooden bed into which vermin have once made their way. Folding beds and lounges even of the best type are unhygienic, usually too low for the patient's comfort, and often insecure.

A bedstead should be wiped frequently with a damp cloth; if it is of enameled iron it may be washed with soap and water. The springs may be cleansed with a stiff brush dipped in kerosene oil. Excessive use of water upon the springs is likely to make them rust.

MATTRESSES.--Various substances are used in the manufacture of mattresses, but nothing has yet been found that is as satisfactory as curled hair. It is light and clean and elastic, it does not readily absorb odors, and it is easily renovated. Although hair is more costly than other materials, a hair mattress may be used almost indefinitely if it is occasionally made over.

Felt or cotton mattresses are firm, but heavy, difficult to keep clean, and likely to absorb odors. A useful mattress made from straw is sometimes found in country districts. Such a bed is thoroughly hygienic, for the worn straw may be burned and the tick washed and refilled with clean straw; but straw beds are generally hard and lumpy. The least desirable of all mattresses is the old fashioned feather bed, and it should never be used if a better can by any possibility be obtained; but a feather bed should not be arbitrarily taken away from an old person accustomed to its use, unless his welfare is really at stake.

A mattress made in two sections is unnecessary for a single bed; indeed, a mattress made in one piece is more easily kept in place if the patient is restless. A good quality of blue and white ticking makes a serviceable cover for both mattress and pillows since its color is not likely to run.

CARE OF THE MATTRESS.--A mattress should be brushed frequently with a whisk broom, especially around the tufts and edges. If a patient is long confined to bed, a fresh one should occasionally be substituted so that the regular mattress may be removed, well brushed, beaten with a carpet beater, and left exposed to the sun and air for a day or two. A mattress that is badly soiled should be sent to a cleaner and made over; it cannot be cleaned properly at home. It is generally possible to remove blood stains, if they have not soaked through the ticking, by applying a thick cream made from raw starch and cold water. When the starch becomes dry it should be brushed away, and the application should be repeated until the stain has disappeared. For the best results the starch should be applied before the stain is dry.

PILLOWS.--One patient can use an almost unlimited number of feather pillows. Some should be soft and others firm, some large and some small; but pillows that are very large and thick are less useful than a greater number of smaller ones. It is well to have several small pillows of varying size and thickness to support different parts of the body.

Hair pillows are often acceptable in warm weather, and they are also desirable for patients with high fever or excessive perspiration. Rubber air pillows are a convenience in traveling and add much to the comfort of a patient when he first goes out in a carriage or motor car, but air pillows are not sufficiently durable for general use.

If a pillow tick becomes soiled, the feathers may be transferred to a clean tick by making an opening about six inches long in the end of each pillow, sewing the ticks together, and then shaking the feathers from one tick to the other. The soiled tick can then be washed. If the feathers themselves have become soiled they should be renovated by a cleaner. Pillows, like mattresses, should be frequently brushed, sunned, and aired. They should not be held in the mouth while a clean pillow-case is adjusted.

PROTECTION OF THE MATTRESS AND PILLOWS.--In all cases of sickness the mattress must be adequately protected. Neglect is inexcusable and may cause expense and trouble as well as discomfort to the patient.

The following may be used to protect the mattress or pillows: large quilted pads, small pads of cotton batting covered with old muslin or cheese cloth, slip covers for the mattress, rubber sheets and pillow-cases, old blankets and quilts that may be washed easily. Heavy wrapping paper, builders' paper, and newspapers serve well in emergencies, or for a short time.

RUBBER SHEETS AND PILLOW-CASES.--Soft rubber cloth, single or double faced, is most frequently used when it is necessary to protect the bed from discharges. It may be purchased by the yard. Rubber sheets should not be used unless they are really necessary. They are hot and uncomfortable, and increase the tendency to perspire. When used, a rubber sheet should be 1 yard wide or wide enough to reach from the lower edge of the pillows down to the patient's knees, and long enough so that it can be tucked in securely on both sides of the bed. Rubber sheets may be cleaned by laying them on a flat surface and washing on both sides with soap and water, using a small brush if necessary. After rinsing they should be wiped, and when thoroughly dry they should be rolled rather than folded, to prevent the rubber from breaking.

Rubber pillow-cases are used for a patient who perspires profusely, or who has a discharge of any kind from the head or neck, and also when substances which may wet or stain the pillow are applied to the head. They should be put on next to the pillow, securely fastened with tapes, snap hooks, or buttons, and covered with the regular pillow slip.

Rubber sheets and pillow-cases are not durable. They should be used carefully, and frequently examined for holes or worn places by holding them up to the light. Even a pin hole near the center may render a rubber sheet or pillow-case as useless as a sieve.

SHEETS.--Sheets of ample proportions are necessary for comfort, and important for sanitary reasons as well. For a bed of the dimensions mentioned in this lesson sheets should be three yards long, and two yards wide. A safe rule for any bed is to have the sheets one yard longer and one yard wider than the mattress. A sheet of these dimensions is large enough to be tucked under the sides and foot of the mattress, while at least twelve inches are left to fold over the blankets at the top. Cotton sheets are as good as linen for general use, or even better, and are far less expensive.

DRAW SHEETS are used to cover rubber sheets, and to protect beds when the rubbers are not used. In hospitals special draw sheets are usually provided, but an ordinary sheet folded answers every purpose. New and expensive sheets should not be used for draw sheets, since they are more likely than other sheets to become stained. Draw sheets should be wide enough to extend about four inches beyond the rubber sheet at the top and bottom.

PILLOW COVERS.--Pillow covers are generally made of cotton, but persons who can afford the cost frequently prefer linen, especially in hot weather. Unless fastened with buttons or tapes, a pillow case should be several inches longer than its pillow. It should be wide enough to slip on easily, but not so wide that it wrinkles or allows the pillow to turn. If it is too small the pillow will become hard and uncomfortable. These small things, unimportant as they are to the well, may cause much discomfort to a restless or nervous patient.

BLANKETS.--All wool blankets are both light and warm, and are consequently the most comfortable bed covering. But unless they can be dry cleaned frequently, it is better to select blankets made from one part wool and two parts cotton. Blankets containing equal parts of wool and cotton are warmer, but are more injured by washing. Very light blankets of wool or outing flannel are useful in summer. Double blankets should always be cut in two and bound at the ends, since single blankets are easier than double blankets to handle and wash. Patients are frequently too warmly covered by day. Too much warmth is enervating, it causes the patient to perspire, and makes him restless and more susceptible to draughts and to changes of temperature. Two light blankets are warmer and more comfortable than one heavy blanket.

COMFORTERS AND QUILTS.--Heavy cotton comforters are burdensome without being correspondingly warm. Eiderdown quilts or those padded with wool are good for a patient who sleeps out of doors, or whose room is kept at a low temperature. Bed covers that cannot be laundered readily should be protected by basting on both sides of the top a wide piece of muslin or linen, which can be removed and washed.

COUNTERPANES.--White dimity counterpanes are desirable, since they are light in weight, easily laundered, and inexpensive. A heavy counterpane is uncomfortable at any time, and still more uncomfortable in sickness. If a light spread is not available, a sheet makes a good substitute. A counterpane should be wide enough to cover the sheets and blankets at the sides when the bed is open, and long enough to protect the bedding at the top and bottom.

BED MAKING

All methods of making beds for the sick are based upon a few underlying principles. The aim in every case is to obtain the following results with the least expenditure of time and labor: first, to secure comfort for the patient, and to eliminate all causes of friction, irritation, or pressure upon his skin; next to keep the covers firmly in place, so that the bed will not easily become disarranged; then to protect the mattress, and last, to secure as good an appearance as possible.

[Illustration: FIG. 12.--THE DRAW SHEET IN PLACE. (*From "Elementary Nursing Procedures," California State Board of Health.*)]

TO MAKE AN UNOCCUPIED BED, proceed as follows: remove the pillows and covers one at a time, and place them on chairs, near an open window if possible. Brush the mattress and then set it up on its ends to air, or turn it back over the foot board. Wipe the bedstead with a damp cloth. Replace the mattress after it has aired, turning it from side to side and from end to end on alternate days. Cover the mattress, unless it is enclosed in a slip cover, with a white quilted pad or an old blanket, and then spread the lower sheet over the mattress, so that the middle fold of the sheet lies upon the center of the mattress in a straight line from the head of the bed to the foot. Tuck the sheet under, first at the top and then at the bottom, drawing it so that it is firm and tight. If the sheet is of proper length tuck fourteen or sixteen inches under at the top, but take care to cover the mattress at the foot also. Next tuck the sheet under at the side, folding its corners to make a neat finish like an envelope. Place the rubber sheet, if it must be used, across the bed, with its upper edge where the lower edge of the pillows will come. A draw sheet somewhat wider than the rubber sheet is needed next; an ordinary sheet, folded once the long way of the sheet, may be used, with the fold toward the head of the bed. Tuck both rubber and draw sheet securely under the mattress at the side. In some cases the rubber sheet may be placed next to the mattress, and covered by the mattress pad and lower sheet. Place the draw sheet as directed, whether the rubber is used or not. After the lower, rubber, and draw sheets have been adjusted on one side of the bed, go to the opposite side, draw them over smoothly, and tuck them under the mattress as tightly as possible.

Next spread the upper sheet over the bed so that its upper edge reaches to the upper edge of the mattress, and its middle crease lies over the middle line of the mattress, and place it right side down, so that the smooth side of the hem will be uppermost when the sheet is turned over the blankets. Place the blankets so that their upper edges lie a little higher than the place where the lower edge of the pillow will come, and tuck them in firmly at the bottom and sides. If the blankets are not long enough to tuck in at the foot, place the lower blanket as directed and the upper blanket five or six inches lower than the first. When tucked in, the upper blanket holds the lower one in place fairly well. Place the counterpane evenly and smoothly, tuck it under at the foot, turn its corners neatly, turn its upper edge under the upper edge of the blankets and fold the upper sheet down over the whole. Last of all, shake the pillows and place them neatly on the bed.

[Illustration: FIG. 13.--THE CLOSED BED. (*From "Elementary Nursing Procedures," California State Board of Health.*)]

Practice is necessary before it is possible to make a bed quickly and well, and a certain amount of proficiency in making an unoccupied bed should be acquired before undertaking to make a bed with a patient in it. One should learn to work in an orderly way, without confusion, unnecessary motion, or jarring of the bed.

TO CHANGE A PATIENT'S PILLOWS.--Stand preferably on the right side of the bed and slip the left arm under the patient's shoulders, supporting his head in the hollow of the arm. Raise him slightly and remove the pillows one at a time with the right hand, drawing them outward on the left side of the bed. Place a small pillow under his head. Shake the pillows, change the cases if necessary, and replace them on the left side of the bed, ready to be drawn back into position. Raise the patient as before, remove the small pillow and draw the others into place. It is sometimes better to hold the patient on the upper pillow while removing and replacing the under one.

LIFTING A PATIENT IN BED.--Patients tend to slip down toward the foot of the bed, and they should be raised if unable to help themselves. To raise the patient, instruct him to flex his knees and to press his feet firmly upon the bed; place one arm under his shoulders, as when changing pillows, the other arm under the thighs, and lift him upward without jerking. The lifting can be done more easily by two people, and with less discomfort to the patient: if he is entirely helpless two people are necessary. Two people should proceed as follows: Let *A* place her left arm under the patient's head and shoulders as before, her right arm under the small of his back; let *B* place her right arm also under the small of his back and her left arm under his thighs, and at a signal let them lift together. In this way the weight is so evenly distributed that a heavy person can be lifted without great difficulty.

TO TURN A PATIENT IN BED.--A patient may be turned toward or away from you. In turning a patient toward you, place one hand over his farther shoulder and the other over his hip, and turn him toward you. Then flex his knees slightly. To turn a patient from you, pass one hand as far as possible under the shoulders, and the other as far as possible under the thighs. Then raising the patient slightly, draw him back toward you, turning him at the same time, and then flex the knees. Lastly place a pillow firmly against his back to support it.

TO CHANGE THE SHEETS WHILE THE PATIENT IS IN BED proceed as follows: First collect the fresh linen and place it conveniently near the bed. Then draw the bedclothes from beneath the mattress, raising the mattress meanwhile with one hand to prevent jarring the bed. Remove first the spread and then the upper blanket if there are two, fold each once and place it on a chair. Hold the remaining blanket in place with one hand, while with the other you draw the upper sheet out from under it; then fold the edges of the blanket up over the patient to keep them out of the way. The upper sheet, unless soiled, may be folded once and used again as a draw sheet. Next remove all the pillows, unless the patient prefers to keep one. Then move the patient toward one side of the bed and turn him on his side so that he faces the edge nearest him. Roll the draw sheet and rubber sheet together if both are to be removed, or separately if the rubber sheet is to remain on the bed; then roll the bottom sheet throughout its entire length, and bring the three sheets, all rolled as flat and as tightly as possible, close to the patient's back. Pleat about half of the fresh lower sheet lengthwise and place the pleated portion as close as possible to the rolled soiled sheets. Tuck in the other half of the fresh sheet at the top, bottom and side, draw the rubber sheet if it is to be replaced back over the fresh lower sheet, arrange the fresh draw sheet in place, tuck it in at the side, and roll its free portion close to the patient's back. The fresh side of the bed is then ready for the patient. Lift his feet back over the rolled sheets keeping his knees flexed, then turn him back over the rolled sheets on to the fresh smooth part, remove the soiled sheets and arrange the fresh ones in place on the side where the patient has just been lying. Be careful to keep him well covered with the blanket. After the lower sheets are in place and firmly tucked in, spread above the blanket the fresh upper sheet, and over the sheet spread the second blanket. Hold the sheet and blanket in place with one hand while using the other hand to draw out the first blanket from beneath the sheet. In this way the patient is constantly covered by a blanket. Place the blanket just removed above the other and finish the bed according to the directions given for an unoccupied bed, using special care, however not to draw the covers too tightly over the patient's feet.

[Illustration: FIG. 14.--CHANGING THE DRAW SHEET. (*From Pope "Home Care of the Sick," American School of Home Economics, Chicago.*)]

TO MOVE A PATIENT FROM ONE BED TO ANOTHER.--On the fresh bed have the lower sheets in place but not the upper covers. Place the two beds close together side by side, and draw one mattress a little over the place where the two sides meet. Loosen the draw sheet under the patient, roll it on both sides close to the body and draw him gently over by means of this sheet, moving his shoulders at the same time. If the beds are unequal in height, use firm pillows or folded blankets to make an inclined plane.

[Illustration: FIG. 15.--CHANGING A PATIENT FROM ONE BED TO ANOTHER. (*From Pope "Home Care of the Sick," American School of Home Economics, Chicago.*)]

If the beds differ greatly in height and indeed in most cases, it is better to carry the patient from one bed to the other. At least two people are needed; one alone should never attempt to carry anyone heavier than a small child. One method for lifting is as follows: Let two bearers, *A* and *B* stand on the same side of the bed. If the patient is to be moved into the right side of the fresh bed let both bearers stand on the right side of the occupied bed; if he is to go into the left side of the fresh bed, let them both stand on the left side of the occupied bed. Let *A* place one arm under the patient's shoulders and her other under the small of his back, while *B* places one arm under his hips and the other just below his knees. Draw the patient to the edge of the bed, instruct him to place his arms about the shoulders of *A* and to hold the body rigid, and then lift together at a given signal, keeping his weight well up on the chests of the bearers.

Whenever a patient must be turned, lifted, carried, or moved in any way, let him know beforehand just what you intend to do so that he may not be startled, and also that he may coöperate if possible. Grasp him firmly but gently, avoid pinching the skin, and move him steadily and smoothly, avoiding jerks and false starts. Do not attempt alone more than your strength is amply sufficient to accomplish, and endeavor at all times to handle the sick with the utmost gentleness and consideration.

EXERCISES

1. Describe a bedstead and mattress suitable for a sick person's use, and tell why they are to be preferred.

2. How should the bedstead be cared for? the mattress? the pillows?

3. How should a mattress and pillows be protected?

4. Describe in detail the bed covers that are desirable for use in sickness.

5. Name the results that a good method of bedmaking aims to secure.

6. Describe the method of making an unoccupied bed.

7. How should one change the pillows of a helpless patient?

8. Describe the way in which you would lift and turn a patient in bed.

9. Describe the method of changing sheets and remaking a bed while the patient is in it.

10. Why are beds and bedmaking considered so important in the care of the sick?

FOR FURTHER READING

Notes on Nursing--Florence Nightingale, Pages 79-84.

CHAPTER VII

BATHS AND BATHING

Bathing is necessary in sickness no less than in health. It stimulates and equalizes the circulation, is soothing in feverish conditions, is refreshing to most people, and by affording a certain amount of exercise it lessens the fatigue of lying in bed. Moreover, without frequent bathing it is impossible to keep the skin in good condition, since scales of dead skin, oily matter, and solid substances left by perspiration collect on the surface of the body when a person is lying still in bed as well as when he is leading an active life. The common belief that sick people are likely to catch cold from bathing is quite unfounded; every patient, unless his condition is such that the doctor orders otherwise, should have one complete cleansing bath each day. In addition to the regular cleansing bath other kinds are often prescribed as medical treatment.

CLEANSING BATHS

A *tub bath* if allowed by a patient's condition, is the most satisfactory kind, but special precautions must be taken to guard her from fatigue and chill. The bath room and everything to be used should be made ready before she leaves her bed. Necessary clothing and toilet articles should be collected and arranged conveniently, a chair covered with a blanket and also a bath mat should be placed beside the tub, and the temperature of the bath room should be regulated so that it is about 70° F., or a little lower if the room is likely to become overheated as the bath proceeds. The bath water should be drawn last. Its temperature, tested by a thermometer, should be between 96° and 100° at the beginning, and may be increased if desirable.

If the patient is weak, wash and dry her face, neck, and ears, and if necessary cut the finger and toe nails before she leaves the bed, in any case before she enters the tub. As soon as the patient has left the bed, strip it and leave it to air; then assist her into the bath room and help her carefully into the tub. Do not allow her to stay in the water more than ten minutes at most, and stop the bath at once if she shows the slightest sign of faintness, dizziness, exhaustion, difficult breathing, marked change of color, or other unusual symptom. Indeed, if the patient is weak or her reaction to the bath uncertain, as when she takes her first tub bath after an illness, someone should always be within call to help the attendant in case of need. A faint, heavy patient in a bath tub is an impossible load for one person to handle.

While the patient is in the tub, soap her well, brush her finger and toe nails, rinse, and rub her to stimulate the circulation. Then help her from the tub, seat her in the chair, draw the blanket closely about her from neck to feet, dry her with warm towels, exposing the body as little as possible, and, if she is to return to bed, put on a fresh night gown, and wrapper and slippers. Next place the lower sheet, the draw sheet, and one pillow on the bed as quickly as possible, help the patient into bed, keeping her well covered with a blanket, and finish making the bed. If she seems chilly, give a hot water bag and hot drink and leave the blanket next her in place. After the patient has been made comfortable, clean the tub and put the bath room in order.

Even patients supposedly able to take tub baths without assistance should not lock the bath room door nor be left alone a long time.

BED BATH.--Practice is essential in order to give a bed bath skillfully. The aim is to make the patient thoroughly clean and thoroughly dry, without chilling, fatiguing, or exposing her, without making the bed damp, and without unnecessary haste or delay. One method of giving a bed bath follows, but any method that accomplishes these aims is likely to be satisfactory.

First see that the room is about 70° F. and likely to remain so, and exclude draughts. Collect everything to be used, including a blanket to cover the patient, an old blanket or large bath towel to protect the bed, at least two other towels, one a bath towel and the other a face towel, two wash cloths, soap, nail brush, powder, alcohol, comb and brush, nail file, scissors, etc.; fresh bed and personal linen; a large basin containing water at 105°, a jug of hotter water, and a slop jar. Remove the upper bed clothes except one blanket, which should cover the patient constantly during the bath, and spread them where they will air; remove all the pillows but one, and place the bath blanket under the patient as the under sheet is placed in bed making. If a bath blanket is not used, keep the bath towel under the part that is being bathed by moving the towel from place to place.

Next remove the night gown in the following way: Let the patient lie on her back, with her knees flexed; draw the gown up as far as possible, then raise or get her to raise her hips so that the gown may be drawn up above the waist. Next raise her head and shoulders with one arm and draw the night gown up to the neck with the other; remove one sleeve, draw the gown over the head and then off the other arm.

[Illustration: FIG. 16.--WASHING A PATIENT WITHOUT EXPOSURE. (*Sanders "Modern Methods in Nursing."*)]

The patient is now ready for the bath. Wet the wash cloth thoroughly, but hold it gathered in the hand so that it will not drip. Wash the face, neck, and ears first, dry them thoroughly, and next, using the second wash cloth, wash the arms and hands, chest and abdomen, giving particular attention to the armpits and navel. Raise the blanket slightly with one hand to keep it from becoming damp, but expose the patient as little as possible; the arms and legs need not remain covered while being washed. Dry each part thoroughly before washing the next. Next turn the patient on her side and wash the back, the buttocks, and upper part of the thighs; give special attention to the fold between the buttocks. Then turn the patient on her back, and wash the thighs, legs, and feet. If it is important to move the patient as little as possible, leave the back until last so that the under sheet may be changed without turning her again. Cut the toe nails if necessary before washing, and clean them carefully afterward. Unless there is a reason to the contrary, wash the hands and the feet in the basin, first protecting the bed with a towel, newspaper, or clean wrapping paper. Be sure to clean well between the toes, and to dry the feet thoroughly; they may need some friction. Throughout the bath empty and refill the basin as necessary.

Wash the genital region last. Let the patient lie upon her back with knees flexed and separated, or upon one side with the knees flexed and one slightly raised. Patients who are able may take this part of the bath themselves with whatever assistance may be necessary. The attendant, however, must either do it herself or make sure that the patient does it thoroughly. To neglect a helpless patient is always unkind, and no less unkind when the motive is a mistaken sense of modesty. If discharge from the genitals is present use absorbent cotton, or clean, soft old cloth to wash the parts, and burn it afterward. It is sometimes desirable to place the patient on a bedpan and rinse the parts by a gentle stream of warm water poured from a jug. After the attendant has completed this part of the bath she should wash her own hands thoroughly.

After the bath rub the patient with alcohol. If a complete alcohol rub is impossible, at least rub the points where pressure comes, especially the back. After the rub apply a little toilet powder if the patient desires it. When the toilet is complete remove the bath blanket, remake the bed and put the room in order.

CARE OF THE MOUTH AND TEETH.--In sickness the mouth and teeth require more than ordinary attention; indeed, the condition of a patient's mouth is a fair index to the quality of the care she is receiving. If the patient can brush her own teeth she should do so in the morning, at night, and after meals. At those times the attendant, without waiting to be asked, should bring her a towel, tooth-brush, cup of tepid water, tooth paste or powder, and a small basin or dish to receive the used water. The process is generally more thorough when the patient does it herself, and even a patient unable to sit up can brush her teeth successfully if the nurse holds the powder and cup of water, and provides a basin shallow enough for the patient to use by turning her head to one side.

[Illustration: FIG. 17.--THE NURSE ASSISTING THE PATIENT IN BRUSHING THE TEETH. (*From "Elementary Nursing Procedures," California State Board of Health.*)]

The attendant must cleanse the mouth of a patient who is unable to do it herself. If this cleansing is neglected, a dark tenacious substance collects upon the teeth and gums, composed chiefly of food particles, bacteria, mouth secretions, and worn out cells of the mucous membrane. Once formed it is difficult to remove, hence the mouths of all patients and especially those who have fever, must receive proper care from the very beginning of illness. Cotton swabs are convenient for cleansing the mouth; they are made by winding a small piece of absorbent cotton upon a match or wooden tooth-pick.

To cleanse the mouth of a helpless patient, take to the bedside the mouth wash prescribed by the doctor, a towel to protect the bedclothes, several swabs, and a receptacle for used swabs; the latter should be a strong paper bag or several thicknesses of newspaper. Clean the tongue, gums, teeth, and spaces between the teeth gently but thoroughly, using especial care if the gums are tender. Dip only clean swabs in the solution, discard each one after using it once, and burn it afterward. Let the patient rinse her mouth after cleansing it if she is strong enough. If the mouth is very dry, encourage her to drink more water. Notify the doctor if the gums and tongue crack or bleed since he may wish to order a special mouth wash. Cold cream or boracic ointment may be used if the lips are dry and cracked.

False teeth should be thoroughly brushed and cleansed, and kept in cold water if taken out during the night.

CARE OF THE HAIR.--Long hair, if neglected, becomes tangled and matted in a surprisingly short time. Unless the patient is actually in a dying condition she is not too sick to have it properly attended to at least once a day. Before combing the hair protect the pillow with a towel; then part the hair in the middle from the forehead to the nape of the neck, and draw it to either side. Begin to comb at the ends, holding the strand of hair firmly in one hand placed between the head and the comb; in this way tangles can be removed without hurting. After combing and brushing the hair, braid it in two braids, beginning near the ears; draw it as tightly or loosely near the head as the patient prefers, but remember that tight braids mean fewer tangles. If the hair is heavy or badly tangled the patient may be too much fatigued to have it all combed at one time; in this case braid the part that has been finished and complete the work later.

TO WASH THE HAIR OF A BED PATIENT.--The hair of a patient can be successfully washed in bed if sufficient care is taken not to chill or tire the patient, or to wet the bed. The following articles are needed: one small jug of strong soap suds made by dissolving a pure soap in hot water, one large jug of hot water at about 112° F., one jug of cold water, a slop jar or foot tub, one long rubber sheet or piece of enamel cloth, and several towels including at least one bath towel. Let the patient lie as near the edge of the bed as possible. Roll one small towel lengthwise, place it below the hair at the back of the neck, bring it up above the ears to the forehead and pin tightly, in order to catch water that might wet the face and neck. Next make a kind of trough of the large rubber by rolling its long edges inward for a few inches. Place this across the bed under the patient's head so that her neck rests on the lower roll. Raise by means of pillows the end of the rubber trough that lies toward the middle of the bed, in order to prevent water from running into the bed or collecting under the patient's head. Let the other end of the rubber extend over the edge of the bed down into the slop jar or foot tub, which may be placed on a chair or stool. Then wash the hair and scalp with the soap solution, and rinse them thoroughly with water from the large jug. Squeeze as much water as possible from the hair, remove the rubber and substitute a heavy bath towel, and rub and fan the hair until dry. A shampoo in bed is tiring. Do not attempt it unless the patient is strong enough to stand not only the shampoo itself, but also a complete change of bed clothing, which will almost certainly be necessary if the attendant has been careless or clumsy in the slightest degree.

HOT FOOT BATHS properly speaking are medical treatment, but they are taken by many persons to relieve colds, headache, or insomnia. Let the patient sit, well wrapped, with her feet in water at about 105°, and then increase the temperature gradually by adding hotter water. Take care to add hot water slowly and not to pour it directly upon the patient's feet or ankles; otherwise she may be scalded. Mustard may be added to the bath water in the proportion of one tablespoonful of mustard to each gallon of water. If mustard is to be used make it into a smooth paste with cold water, thin the paste with warm water, and when thin enough to pour easily add it to the bath water and stir well. The bath may continue for 10 to 20 minutes, and the feet should be dried afterward without friction. The patient should go to bed at once; she should not wander about, clearing away her foot bath, doing forgotten things, getting herself chilled, and losing all the good effects.

A foot bath may be given easily to a patient in bed. Bring to the bedside a blanket, a towel, the tub filled with water, and something with which to protect the bed; this may be a rubber sheet, bath towel, old blanket folded, or several thick clean newspapers. Loosen the upper covers at the foot of the bed, fold them back above the patient's knees, and cover her legs and feet with the extra blanket making it overlap the bed clothing so that it will not slip. Flex the patient's knees, put the bed protector under her feet, place the tub on the side of the bed, raise the legs and feet with one hand and arm, and slide the tub into place with the other, raising the elbow in such a way that it keeps the blanket out of the water. Lower the feet slowly into the water, fold the towel, and place it over the edge of the tub in order to protect the patient's knees from the cold rim; then tuck the blanket closely about the tub and legs and proceed as before. After the bath use the towel, unless it is wet, to receive the feet when they are withdrawn from the tub. Remove the tub, dry the feet thoroughly, cover them warmly, and remake the bed.

COOL SPONGE BATH.--For feverish patients doctors often order cool sponge baths. In order to give a cool sponge bath, first protect the bed thoroughly, but leave the patient uncovered except for a towel laid over the hips. Use cool water, or cool water and alcohol, and have the wash cloth as wet as it can be without dripping. Bathe the body without friction, using long, light strokes, and leave each part wet until the bath has been completed. Do not use soap. Sponge in this way the arms, legs, chest, and back, but not the abdomen, for ten to twenty minutes, giving special attention to the neck and inner side of the arms and legs, because in those places large blood vessels lie nearer the surface of the body. After finishing the bath dry the body by patting it gently with towels.

Take the patient's pulse occasionally during the bath, and stop the bath at once if the patient's pulse grows weaker, if she shivers violently, or if her face, fingers, or toes turn a bluish color. Babies react rapidly to cool sponging; for a baby use tepid water, sponge for five minutes only, and watch the child closely during the bath.

EXERCISES

1. What may a bath be expected to accomplish in addition to cleansing?

2. In giving a tub bath, what precautions should be taken to avoid chilling the patient? to avoid tiring the patient?

3. What symptoms would lead you to think that a tub bath was not agreeing with a patient? What should you do in such a case?

4. Name six essentials of a skillfully given bed bath.

5. What preparations should be made and what articles assembled before beginning a bed bath?

6. Describe the method of bathing a patient in bed.

7. What care should the mouth and teeth of every sick person receive? How should such care be given to a patient who is helpless?

8. Describe the daily care of a patient's hair, and tell how a shampoo may be given to a patient in bed.

9. How should you give a mustard foot bath to a patient in bed?

10. When and how should you give a cool sponge bath?

FOR FURTHER READING

The Human Mechanism--Hough and Sedgwick, Chapter XI.

CHAPTER VIII

APPLIANCES AND METHODS FOR THE SICK-ROOM

Patients who are confined to bed even for a few days often suffer acutely from muscular tension, from pressure, and from fatigue due to lack of exercise. Indeed, many a sick person is surprised to find that the bed which had seemed so infinitely desirable can change into a place of torment after a few short days of illness. "Bed-weariness" is hard to bear in any case of illness, but it is doubly hard for persons who are really helpless.

Unless the patient is an experienced sufferer he often has no idea what should be done to make him comfortable; while an equally inexperienced helper, though full of good will, is often discouraged to find that the arrangement she had thought perfect soon fails to satisfy her restless patient. But if she is willing to devote thought and ingenuity to removing small annoyances, she can do many things to alleviate his misery.

BED SORES, or pressure sores, are caused by continued pressure upon the skin. The weight of the body, or of a part of the body, if it comes for a long time upon one place finally interferes with the circulation in the tissues on which the part rests, and consequently interferes with the nutrition of the affected part. Any tissue to which the blood is not bringing all its necessary food supply tends to lose its tone, to become weak, and if the condition persists, to break down altogether.

The direct cause of bed sores then is pressure, and pressure is aggravated by moisture, wrinkles in the bed clothes, crumbs or other hard particles, lack of cleanliness, friction of any kind, or by rough, careless handling. Bed sores occur most often over bony prominences, such as the end of the spine, elbows, heels, shoulders, hips, ankles, and knees, but they may form anywhere, even on the ears or back of the head. They are more likely to appear on thin, aged, or depleted patients. These painful and serious sores can be prevented almost always by faithful care. When they occur, they result in the great majority of cases purely from negligence, and a person who knows the danger and yet through carelessness allows one to develop upon a patient may justly feel herself disgraced.

Prevention of bed sores depends upon keeping the skin dry and clean and upon relieving pressure by special devices and by turning the patient frequently. The parts where pressure comes should be washed at least twice daily with warm water and soap, rubbed frequently with alcohol to improve the circulation and to keep up the tone of the skin, and powdered with a little good toilet powder. Much powder is likely to do harm by collecting in hard, irritating particles. The bed should be kept constantly dry and smooth, and free from crumbs, lumps, wrinkles, or other inequalities. Prolonged pressure should be relieved by turning the patient often,--once every waking hour is not too often if the body is emaciated,--and by pillows, pads, and rings.

Small pillows or thick pads of cotton should be placed under the patient's back and shoulders, between the knees and ankles when he lies on his side, and in other places where sores are likely to develop. Rubber rings are useful, but few patients like them for a long time. They should not be inflated more than necessary to raise the affected part from the bed; if much inflated, they are uncomfortable and may do harm. The ring may be covered with a muslin pillow case, or it may be wound smoothly with long strips of bandage or old muslin. Ordinary cotton batting wound with strips of muslin may be made into rings and used to remove pressure from heels, elbows, or other parts. These cotton rings are less heating than pads, and give better support.

The first sign of a bed sore is either redness of the skin or a dark discoloration like a bruise. Every point where a bed sore may form should be inspected daily. If the slightest symptom of a sore appears, the patient must not lie on the affected part, and every effort should be made to keep the skin from breaking; vigorous rubbing at this stage is dangerous, and will by no means make up for previous neglect. The condition should be reported to the doctor at once. If in spite of all efforts the skin does break, a peculiarly difficult kind of open wound results which must be treated and dressed according to the doctor's directions.

DEVICES TO GIVE SUPPORT.--The variety and number of pillows one patient can use is almost unlimited. A weak patient when lying on his side should have his back supported by a pillow. When he lies on his back a pillow should be placed under his knees to lessen muscular tension, and if he may be raised in bed, several pillows are needed to support him comfortably. A back rest is useful for a patient who can sit up in bed. Satisfactory back rests of several types can be purchased, or one may be improvised from a straight chair placed on the bed bottom side up, so that its legs lie against the head of the bed and its back forms an inclined plane. Back rest and chair alike should be covered by several pillows to make them comfortable, and other pillows should be used to support the patient's arms.

A person who is sitting up in bed always tends to slip down toward the foot. This tendency may be corrected by using a foot rest, knee pad, or pillow. A hard pillow may be placed in the bed at the foot for the patient to brace his feet against; or a short board, well padded, may be arranged as follows for the feet to rest against: Fasten ropes to the board, as the ropes of a swing are fastened to the seat; set the padded board on edge at a convenient point below the patient's feet, and hold it in place by tying the ropes of the "swing" to the head of the bed. A pillow may be used in the same way, either at the feet or under the knees, by folding it over a long strip of muslin, the ends of which are then tied to the sides of the bed, brought up to the head, and there tied to prevent slipping. A cylindrical cushion six or eight inches in diameter and as long as an ordinary pillow, stuffed with firm material, may also be used for this purpose. It should be held in place by strips of strong muslin or ticking sewed to the ends of the cushion and tied to the head of the bed. The cushion should have a washable cover.

[Illustration: FIG. 18.--SHOWING FOOT-SLING FOR SUPPORTING PATIENT IN THE UPRIGHT POSITION. (*Sanders "Modern Methods in Nursing."*)]

Supports called *bed cradles* are used to keep the weight of the bed covers from sensitive parts of the body, generally the feet or abdomen. They are semi-circular pieces of wood or iron fastened together so that they will stand up. A satisfactory cradle may be improvised as follows: Cut a barrel hoop in two, cross the halves at right angles and tie them together firmly; place the cradle over the affected part under the bed clothes. A smaller cradle may be made by taking sections that are less than half of the barrel hoop. If used for one foot only, the cradle should be small enough not to interfere with the motion of the other foot; if used for both feet, it should be large enough to allow some freedom of motion. Since the cradle leaves an air space, the feet should be wrapped in a piece of soft flannel. A cradle used for the protection of the abdomen should extend a little beyond the body on each side.

[Illustration: FIG. 19.--ADJUSTABLE BED REST.]

Adjustable tables are convenient for patients who are able to sit up in bed. These tables are supported on one side only so that they may extend over the bed. Another kind of bedside table has short legs and stands directly on the bed. Such a table can easily be made at home from a wide board with supports six or eight inches high nailed to each end. A lap board supported by heavy books may serve for temporary use. Indeed, home-made substitutes are often as good as expensive apparatus or even better. If sick-room appliances must be bought, it is well to remember that simple standard designs are best. Complicated apparatus is soon out of order, and is generally a trial both to the patient and to those who must adjust it. Persons taking care of chronic patients may often obtain valuable suggestions in regard to appliances by consulting a visiting nurse or the superintendent of the local hospital.

[Illustration: FIG. 20.--ADJUSTABLE TABLE.]

BEDPANS are utensils to receive bowel and bladder discharges of patients lying in bed. Enamel bedpans are better than porcelain, although more expensive. The shape known as the "Perfection" is best for general use. A "slipper" bedpan, although harder to clean and ordinarily less comfortable, may be preferable if it is especially difficult or undesirable to raise the patient. The square or douche pan is preferred by some people, and is especially useful when the quantity of discharge is large, as after an injection.

When a patient asks for the bedpan it should be brought if possible without a moment's delay, not only because no other form of neglect makes a patient realize her helplessness more acutely, but also because the desire to use it often passes quickly and delay may encourage the habit of constipation. If the patient does not ask for the bedpan, the attendant should offer it at suitable times. Bedpans should be warmed before use. An easy way to warm one is to let hot water run over it; the outside should afterward be dried.

To place the bedpan, first flex the patient's knees and push the night gown up; place one hand under the patient's hips, raise them slightly, and with the other hand slip the pan into place. If the patient is entirely helpless two persons are needed to lift her. Place a pad or folded cloth between the patient's back and the pan; then lower the patient gently. Before removing the pan, bring toilet paper, water and two pieces of soft old muslin or gauze. A patient, if able, prefers to use the toilet paper without assistance; her hands should afterward be thoroughly washed. If she is unable, the attendant must do everything needed. After the patient has been cleaned as thoroughly as possible with paper raise her hips with one hand and then remove the pan; it is important to raise her first because the skin often adheres and may be injured if the pan is suddenly pulled away; carelessness in managing the bedpan has caused more than one bed sore. Then remove the pan with one hand and cover at once. Turn the patient, if helpless, on her side, wash the parts with one piece of old muslin, thoroughly dry them with the other, and either burn or thoroughly wash both pieces afterward.

Empty the bedpan and clean it at once; ordinarily one can clean it without wetting or soiling the hands. Use cold water first, removing all adhering solid particles with a tightly rolled piece of toilet paper. Do not use a brush for this purpose. After using cold water, rinse the pan thoroughly in hot water, and at least once a day wash it well in hot soapsuds. Directions for disinfecting the pan will be given later, but remember that a properly kept pan needs no deodorant solution. Glass urinals should be provided for men, and kept clean in the same way. Contents of both bedpan and urinal should always be carefully inspected; neither should be emptied in the dark.

DAILY ROUTINE IN THE SICK-ROOM

Obviously the routine of a patient's day must vary according to her condition, her preferences, and the amount of time the attendant has to give her. The temperature, pulse, and respiration must be taken and all medicine, nourishment, and treatment given at the exact times ordered, but the attendant should learn whether or not the doctor wishes her to wake the patient for food or treatment. Good management in the sick-room depends upon foresight and planning, and therefore it is well to keep in mind the following suggestions:

Vitality is lowest in the early morning, hence baths and treatments, especially if they are fatiguing or painful, should if possible be left until after breakfast. Patients often wake early and wait, weak and miserable, for the day to begin. A hot drink at this time may give relief and enable the patient to sleep again. Even though breakfast time is near, nourishment should be given as soon as the patient wakes. She may not admit that she is hungry, but her nourishment should not be delayed until the family breakfast is ready, or still worse, finished.

Before breakfast the bedpan should be offered, the patient's face and hands should be washed, her teeth brushed, her hair tidied, the bed straightened, and the room put in order. These services should require a few minutes only. The room if properly arranged at bed time needs only a little attention now unless untidy work has gone on during the night; disorder in a sick-room is as unnecessary in the early morning as at any other time.

After the patient has finished her breakfast she may rest, or if allowed, read her mail or the newspaper while the attendant prepares for her day's work; about an hour after breakfast the patient should be bathed, unless she prefers her bath in the evening. After the bath some form of light nourishment should be given, even to a patient who has regular meals. If a patient is able to sit up in a chair, the best time for her to do so is generally just after the bath and toilet have been completed; but if she feels tired she had better wait until afternoon. The bed room can be better aired and cleaned if it is possible to take her into another room; and she herself generally profits by a change of scene.

The doctor should definitely state when and for how long a patient may sit up for the first time after an illness, and an amateur who may be ignorant of the dangers involved should not assume the responsibility of deciding. When a patient is to sit up for the first time, put on her stockings, slippers, and wrapper before she leaves the bed. Arrange an arm chair with pillows in the seat and at the back, bring it close to the bedside and cover it with a large blanket unfolded. The chair may face either the head or the foot of the bed. Help the patient to a sitting position on the extreme edge of the bed, with her feet hanging down. Next, standing in front of her and supporting her well, let her slip down until she stands upon her feet, then let her turn, and gently lower her into the chair. See that the patient while sitting up is warmly covered, and that her foot-stool, pillows, etc., are adjusted comfortably. Move her chair so that the outlook may be as interesting as possible, and at least a little different from the view from the bed. Most patients like to look out of the window; children and old people enjoy it particularly.

If the patient shows signs of fatigue, she should go back to bed even before the appointed time. To help her back to bed, reverse the process of helping her out. A footstool may be needed if the bed is high, or two people to lift her if she is weak or heavy. When a patient is in bed no one should ever sit on the bed, lean against it, use it as a table for folding linen, making pads, etc., take hold of the bed posts in passing, or touch the bed unnecessarily in any way.

The best time for visitors is the last of the morning or the early afternoon. A judicious visitor may do an immense amount of good, especially to a chronic patient; indeed, she may be the only ray of light in a dark day. Subjects of conversation should be pleasant, but not too stimulating or exciting. The visitor should be prepared to carry the burden of the conversation, to drop topics skillfully that seem to involve fatigue or excitement, and either to go or to stop talking if the patient seems tired. Visitors should remember to talk naturally and cheerfully on ordinary topics, and to avoid excessive sympathy and labored attempts to cheer the patient. They should also remember that few patients bear well even the mildest forms of teasing. The patient's room is not the place to discuss personal or family troubles; yet it is only too often chosen for such purposes, probably because the complainer knows that in it an audience is always to be found.

Visitors not belonging to the family should not be present in the sick-room during treatment of any kind, unless their help is required; neither, as a rule, should they stay during the patient's meals. A member of the family may stay with advantage if the patient tires of eating alone, but casual visitors almost invariably offend by undue urging if the patient's appetite is poor, or by facetious remarks if it is good.

Ordinarily only one visitor should be admitted at a time, since a weak patient may be tired merely by looking from one to another. If it is desirable to limit the call, the attendant should tell the visitor beforehand how long to stay, or arrange a signal for the visit to end. To announce baldly in the sick-room that the patient is tired and the visitor must go, will only elicit aggrieved protests from both. In illness lasting only a day or two all visitors should be discouraged; during colds, because they are communicable; during general fatigue, headaches, digestive upsets, and painful menstruation, because rest and quiet are highly desirable. Visitors at such times too frequently give injudicious sympathy, and may actually delay the recovery of patients who enjoy playing the rôle of interesting invalid.

The time when a trustworthy visitor is present may be the best time for the attendant to rest. The patient should be told when the attendant is going, and approximately when she will return. It is a mistake to slip away while the patient sleeps; she seldom fails to wake before the time scheduled and to resent the desertion. Surprises of any kind, pleasant or unpleasant, are seldom good for patients.

Toward the end of the afternoon the patient is probably tired, especially if she has not slept during the day. When fever is present her headache and restlessness increase as the day goes on, but it should be remembered that uncomfortable beds and too heavy covers cause much of the restlessness attributed to fever. Rubbing the back and legs with alcohol, giving a tepid sponge bath, remaking the bed or changing her position may help to soothe her.

The evening should be kept free from excitement, and every possible effort should be made to encourage sleep. It is a mistake to think that a better night results from keeping a sleepy patient awake all the evening; sick people should sleep when they can. Just before bedtime the attendant should prepare her own cot, and then make the following preparations for the patient to sleep: wash the patient's face and hands or give a sponge bath if it is desired, brush the hair, change the night gown, brush crumbs from the bed, tighten the sheets or remake the bed if necessary, rub the back and other pressure points with alcohol, shake the pillows, give liquid nourishment, preferably hot, cleanse the mouth, and give the bedpan. See that the patient's feet are warm, the bed covers right, the room ventilated properly and in good order, and the light extinguished or arranged for the night. If the patient is inclined to be wakeful a hot foot bath may help her, or sponging the entire length of the spine for fifteen minutes, using very hot water and long downward quiet strokes. No conversation should be encouraged during preparations for the night. Patients in bed all day often lose the habit of sleeping at the regular time, and lie awake far into the night from a vague feeling that someone else is coming or something further is to be done for them. Consequently last of all ask the patient if she wants anything more; if not, say good-night, go out and stay out, at least until she has had a chance to go to sleep. She is thus helped to realize that nothing further is likely to happen, and that it is time to go to sleep.

Toward morning the patient grows weaker. More bed covers will probably be needed, and they may often be added without waking her. Night at the best is a dreary time for the sick. Pain and weariness and discouragement are less bearable in the darkness; nervous fears and morbid fancies defy control. Never is kindness more needed or more appreciated than it is by those who lie awake and watch for the morning.

EXERCISES

1. Name all the causes, direct and indirect, of pressure sores.

2. Why are pressure sores generally more serious than injuries of equal extent to the skin of a well person?

3. Where are pressure sores most likely to occur and what are their symptoms?

4. What measures should be employed to prevent pressure sores?

5. Describe ways to support a person lying down in bed.

6. Describe ways to support a person sitting up in bed.

7. How may the weight of the bedclothes be removed from any particular part of the body?

8. How should a bedpan be cared for?

9. Describe in detail a day's routine either of yourself the last time you were ill in bed, or of another patient personally known to you. Could the plan of the day have been improved, and if so, in what ways?

CHAPTER IX

FEEDING THE SICK

Substances used for food are generally grouped into three classes, called the three nutrients. The nutrients are: first, the proteids or nitrogenous substances, which are found in meat, fish, eggs, milk, cheese, peas, beans, etc.; second, the carbohydrates, which include sugars and starch; and third, the fats, which are found in butter, oil, the fat of meat, etc. In addition to the nutrients, water and certain mineral salts are essential to life, while some indigestible material like the fibre of vegetables is needed to give bulk and to stimulate the action of the intestines.

The nutrients furnish the body with materials for growth, and for repair of tissues worn out by use; they also furnish fuel substances from which the body obtains its heat and its energy. All three nutrients can serve as fuel, but the proteids alone can furnish materials for growth and repair of tissues. In order to be used by the body for any purpose, nutrients must first go through a series of complicated changes known as digestion, which renders them soluble so that they can soak through the walls of the intestine.

THE DIGESTIVE PROCESS

Digestion begins in the mouth. There the food is crushed and its fibres separated by the teeth, it is moistened by the saliva, and substances in the saliva begin a chemical action upon the starch. Chewing should be sufficient to reduce the food to a soft mass well moistened with saliva. Slow eating is desirable, but the emphasis should be placed on thorough chewing. For instance, long intervals between bites are of no special benefit if mouthfuls of food are washed down by swallows of water.

After it has been swallowed, the food passes into the stomach and remains there for a variable length of time, while it undergoes further preparation for absorption. It is moved about by the contraction of the muscular walls of the stomach, so that it becomes mixed with the stomach juices and more thoroughly softened. Some digestion of proteids goes on in the stomach, and a little absorption through the walls.

Little by little the food is discharged from the stomach into the small intestine, and the most important part of digestion then begins. It is acted upon chemically by a fluid flowing into the intestine from an organ called the pancreas; this pancreatic juice acts upon all three nutrients and is of great importance in the digestive process. The bile and other juices that flow into the intestine perform important functions also.

The food masses are moved along by rhythmic contractions of the intestine, and absorption goes on when the food has been so changed that it can soak through the intestinal walls into the blood and lymph vessels. The small intestine is about 20 feet long, and consequently affords a large surface for absorption, as does also the large intestine, into which the small intestine opens. The blood and lymph carry the digested food substances to all parts of the body, and thus the different tissues are provided with the materials they need for growth, repair, and energy. Excess of food substances may be stored as fat or expelled from the body.

As the blood and lymph go through the tissues they take from the tissues the refuse, or the part that remains after the fuel substances have been consumed. This refuse from the tissues may be likened to the ashes from a furnace; it is finally eliminated from the body through the kidneys and lungs, and to some extent through the skin and bowels. The part of the food that is not digested of course never soaks through the intestinal walls; it merely passes through the small and large intestines and is finally expelled as feces or bowel movements. The characteristic odor of fecal matter results from the action of bacteria upon it while in the large intestine.

It must be remembered that the body is not nourished merely by swallowing food: in order to nourish the body food must also be digested, absorbed, and made use of by the tissues. Many factors may operate both in health and in sickness to render food indigestible. It may be originally unsuited to the human digestive apparatus, or spoiled, or poor in quality, or badly cooked. But even when wholesome in itself it may be ill-adapted to a particular person at a particular time; thus it may be too great in amount, or eaten at improper hours. Moreover a person's own idiosyncrasy or manner of living or fatigue or illness may render it especially indigestible for him.

Experiments have shown that pain, fear, worry, and other unpleasant emotions actually stop the action of the digestive juices and check muscular contractions of the small intestine. Furthermore, even the absence of pleasant anticipation of food has been shown to delay digestion for hours. Thus scientific knowledge confirms our common experience that such mental states seriously interfere with digestion. The converse is also true. Agreeable taste and odor of food, or even pleasurable thought of it, start the secretion of digestive fluids. It is a common saying that the mouth waters at the prospect of inviting food, but it is less well known that appetizing food does actually start the stomach juices also. A person who understands the physiological effect that the emotions have upon digestion is in a far better frame of mind to cope successfully with the difficulties of feeding the sick than one who considers sick persons' likes and dislikes entirely irrational.

FEEDING THE SICK

Nourishing the sick is not always an easy problem, but its importance can hardly be overestimated. Indeed, proper feeding in many illnesses makes the difference between life and death. The actual amount of nourishment needed in sickness is often less than in health, but it may be just as great, or even greater if the illness causes increased tissue waste. Yet the digestive process of a sick person must be rendered as little laborious as possible, all foods ordinarily difficult to digest must be eliminated, certain others must be withheld or restricted according to the nature of the sickness, and in addition one may have to deal with an appetite that is capricious, diminished, or totally absent.

Diet for the sick is often a part of medical treatment; in such cases the doctor will prescribe special diets and his orders must be carefully carried out. Except for special diets, food for the sick is generally divided into four classes: first, liquid or fluid diet; second, semi-solid diet; third, light or convalescent diet; and lastly, full diet. These diets are not very sharply distinguished.

LIQUID DIET generally includes milk, eggnog, albumen water, broths, soup, beef juice, thin gruel, and beverages. Liquid diet makes least demand upon the digestive powers, because it consists of food already dissolved and therefore nearer the condition in which it can be absorbed. Moreover, it is less likely than other foods to contain excess of fat, improperly cooked starches, and other indigestible material. Liquids must be given at regular intervals and at shorter intervals than solid foods; 6 to 8 ounces every two or three hours is not too much if the patient can take it. The doctor usually specifies the amount and the interval. Some patients will take more nourishment at one time if the interval is slightly increased.

SEMI-SOLID DIET includes all fluids and in addition soft milk toast, soft cooked eggs, well cooked cereal, custards, ice cream and ices, junket, and gelatine jellies. Liquid or semi-solid diet is commonly given in acute fevers because digestive juices and other fluids of the body are then diminished, and also because their digestion places a minimum of work upon a system already burdened with bacterial poisons.

LIGHT OR CONVALESCENT DIET generally means a simple mixed diet. In addition to the articles in the two preceding diets it includes oysters, chicken, baked potatoes, most fruits except bananas, simple desserts, white fish, and other meats and vegetables added judiciously until full diet is reached. Fried foods should not be included.

FULL DIET means an unrestricted menu, but even from full diets especially indigestible foods should be excluded. The principles of feeding sedentary persons as described in manuals of dietetics apply to patients who are obliged to be inactive although not really ill, as for example, a patient suffering from a broken leg. Ordinarily in such cases, as in other kinds of illness, the appetite is greatly diminished, but a word of warning should be given against overfeeding patients whose meals are their chief interest. Such patients are only too likely to interpret full diet as anything they desire in any quantity at any time of day or night, and then to attribute their discomfort and irritability to their illness rather than to overeating.

Constipation is especially stubborn in sickness, since the patient is deprived of his usual exercise and variety of food. So far as possible the bowels should be regulated by diet. Laxative foods include most vegetables with a large amount of fibre, coarse cereals and flour, oils and fats, and most fruits and fruit juices. Unfortunately many laxative foods are difficult for sick persons to digest and must therefore be used with caution. A glass of hot or cold water or orange juice an hour before breakfast may be helpful, and at bed time hot lemonade, oranges, prunes, figs, or other fruit if allowed.

It is essential for patients to drink water freely, and it should be given between meals and also between liquid nourishments. Persons inexperienced in the care of the sick frequently make the mistake of bringing water only when a patient asks for it.

Many acute illnesses begin with fever, headache, sore throat, and especially among children with vomiting, diarrhoea, and other digestive disturbances. In such cases all food should be withheld until the doctor comes, but boiled water, hot or cold, should be given freely. Efforts to tempt the appetite are then mistaken; few people are injured and many are benefited by omitting food even for 24 hours at the beginning of an acute illness, and with few exceptions a doctor can be found in a shorter time.

SERVING FOOD FOR THE SICK.--Food for the sick should always be most carefully prepared and of the best quality, and in addition it should be as inviting, as varied, and as well served as possible. Neglect in these respects is inexcusable. Even slight carelessness in preparing or serving food may arouse disgust and thus banish permanently some valuable article from the dietary.

Trays, dishes, tray cloths, and napkins for the patient must be absolutely clean and as attractive as possible. Cracked or chipped dishes should not be used. Individual sets of dishes for the sick may be purchased, and their convenience makes them well worth their price. Paper napkins may be used in many cases to save laundry work; clean white paper is always superior to soiled linen.

Before the tray is brought to the bedside, everything should be arranged so that the patient can eat in comfort. It is bad management to let the soup cool while the patient's pillows and table are being adjusted. In setting the tray great care should be devoted to placing the articles conveniently, and to the appearance and garnishing of the food. Careful serving requires more thought, but little if any more actual time than slovenly serving. Dishes should not be so full that food is spilled in transit; hot dishes should be covered; hot dishes should reach the patient hot, and cold dishes cold. Liquid nourishment in a glass or cup should be served on a small tray or plate covered with a doily. Neither glass nor cup should be held by the rim.

It is not uncommon to overload trays and to serve everything at once in order to save steps, but a patient is ordinarily more interested in a meal that is served in courses unless very long intervals elapse between. Moreover, if the meal is served in courses he is not tempted to eat dessert first and then to refuse the rest of the meal. If food is given sufficiently often it is safer to err on the side of serving too little at a time rather than too much, since the sight of large amounts of food is often disgusting.

The patient's likes and dislikes should be considered as far as possible, but most patients should not be consulted about their menus beforehand. Great variety in one meal is not necessary; it should be introduced by varying successive meals. An article that has been especially disliked should not be served a second time, unless it can be disguised beyond a possibility of detection. An article of food to which a patient objects should be removed at once; one may appear disappointed if it seems wise, but should never argue. When patients persistently refuse necessary nourishment a difficult situation is presented; persuasion and every form of ingenuity must be used, and the doctor's coöperation enlisted. When, for example, a strict milk diet is ordered for a patient who announces that he never takes milk in any circumstances the situation may seem hopeless but it is not necessarily so.

TO FEED A HELPLESS PATIENT.--Helpless and weak patients must be assisted to eat or drink. A napkin should first be placed under the patient's chin. The attendant should place her hand under the pillow, raise the head slightly, and hold the glass to his lips with her other hand. An ordinary tumbler can be used by a patient lying down if it is not more than a quarter full, or a special feeding cup may be purchased. Bent glass tubes may be used for cool liquids; they should be washed immediately after use. A child who can sit up sometimes takes more nourishment if it is given through a soda water straw.

If the patient must be fed with a spoon care should be taken that the liquid is not too hot, but the attendant should not blow upon it to cool it. It should be given from the point of a spoon placed at right angles to the lips, and plenty of time between mouthfuls should be allowed. A swallow should not be given at the moment when the patient is drawing the breath in. Great patience is required if a helpless person is to be fed acceptably. The attendant should sit by the bedside rather than stand, should present at least the appearance of having unlimited time, and should endeavor not to deprive the patient in any way of the satisfaction he may derive from his nourishment.

EXERCISES

1. What needs of the body do food substances supply?

2. Give an outline of the digestive process.

3. Describe the effect of different mental states upon digestion, and give examples of the ways by which a knowledge of these effects may be utilized in feeding patients.

4. Why is the problem of nourishing the body of especial importance in sickness?

5. Name the four ordinary classes of diet for the sick, and mention all the articles you can belonging to each class.

6. Why is constipation a common ailment among patients confined to bed, and what attempts should be made to overcome it by the diet?

7. Why is it necessary for sick persons to drink water freely, and what efforts should the attendant make to encourage them to do so?

8. Describe the proper serving of a patient's tray.

9. How should helpless patients be assisted to eat?

FOR FURTHER READING

Health and Disease--Roger I. Lee, Chapter II.

The Human Mechanism--Hough and Sedgwick, Chapters VIII, XIII, XIX.

Notes on Nursing--Florence Nightingale, Pages 63-79.

How to Live--Fisher and Fisk, Chapter II.

Bodily Changes in Pain, Hunger, Fear and Rage--Cannon, Chapter I.

Food for the Invalid and the Convalescent--Winifred S. Gibbs.

Practical Dietetics--Pattee, Chapters IV, V.

Feeding the Family--Rose.

Diet in Health and Disease--Friedenwald and Ruhrah.

Feeding Children from Two to Seven Years Old--New York City Department of Health.

American Red Cross Text Book on Home Dietetics--Ada Z. Fish.

Emergency Cooking--Pamphlet 708, American Red Cross.

War Diet in the Home--Pamphlet 706, American Red Cross.

Red Cross Conservation Food Course for Children and Special Classes--Pamphlet 705, American Red Cross.

CHAPTER X

MEDICINES AND OTHER REMEDIES

ACTION OF DRUGS.--Modern medical practice increasingly emphasizes diet, baths, exercises, and other hygienic measures in the treatment of sickness. Drugs are given far less than they were a generation ago; yet medicines are still the most familiar of all remedies, and the most abused by those who persist in treating themselves. Misuse of medicine even by intelligent people is astonishingly common.

Problems of sickness and health would be enormously clarified if the uses and limitations of drugs were more generally understood. Many people still believe that every disease can be cured by a drug if only the doctor is clever or lucky enough to think of the right one to give. Such beliefs result naturally enough from centuries of faith in charms and magic, and occasionally are confirmed by remarkable cures apparently brought about by drugs, but really pure coincidence or the result of suggestion.

It is a fact that a few medicines are known which if rightly used actually do cure certain diseases. An example of their action is the curative effect of quinine in malaria. Such medicines, unfortunately, are few. In the great majority of cases medicines do not cure disease; their beneficial action is ordinarily indirect and is due to their power either to increase or to check certain processes within the body.

It is here that the abuse of drugs comes in. Disordered bodily processes give rise to symptoms of disease; and it is the symptoms of disease, not the disease itself, that trouble the patient. A patient with typhoid, for example, is not conscious of the toxins in his blood, but of headache, weakness, and fever; the man with eyestrain is not aware of an imperfectly shaped lens, but of headache and indigestion. What the patient wants is to have his symptoms relieved; in some cases they can be controlled by drugs, and the sufferer then considers himself cured. But the original condition persists: it may in the meantime be improving, but it may on the other hand be growing worse.

Not infrequently it is best to check symptoms, and to check them by means of drugs. When they should be checked, only a thoroughly trained physician is qualified to decide. The question is not one for amateurs, since the whole practice of medicine, including the prescription of drugs, constantly becomes more nearly an exact science. People should obtain and follow expert advice in regard to health as they would in regard to other affairs of life. The constant self-dosing practised by thousands of people is harmful and unintelligent; it is, however, no less irrational to go to the other extreme and refuse to take medicine prescribed by a competent doctor.

AMATEUR DOSING.--Amateur dosing either of oneself or of others is dangerous in more ways than one. In the first place, time is lost. Moreover, symptoms are characteristic; checking or altering them increases the difficulty of finding the real trouble. The man with eyestrain who takes one drug to stop his headache and another to "cure" his stomach, is simply delaying the time when properly adjusted glasses will relieve both. In this case the result may not be serious; but such a loss of time in finding the trouble and beginning proper treatment might prove fatal in the case of tuberculosis.

Another objection to amateur prescription of medicine is the fact that most drugs have more than one effect. In addition to their main action they have others, subordinate or ordinarily less marked. These minor effects may be serious in some cases. Many headache remedies, for example, affect the heart; a dose that is harmless for a normal person may be strong enough to injure seriously a person with a weak heart. A doctor, and a doctor only, is competent to decide when and in what quantity medicines will be beneficial, because he alone understands both the condition of the patient and all the possible effects of the drug.

In no circumstances should medicine prescribed for one person be taken by another. This rule seems obvious enough; yet every day people pass on their pet remedies to friends. Some medicines deteriorate after standing, and others grow stronger; nevertheless, medicine supposed to have cured a cough or a tonic supposed to have strengthened some member of the family after an attack of grippe is cheerfully administered months later to another member of the family, who, to make matters worse, may differ in age, strength, and probably in the nature of his sickness. Drugs are expensive, and it is considered economical to use them up; measured by lost time and impaired health such practices may be anything but thrifty.

Cathartics, tonics, and various drugs to relieve pain and sleeplessness are among the remedies most commonly taken without medical advice. Enough has already been said about constipation to indicate proper hygienic treatment, but another warning should be given against habitual use of cathartics. Many of these drugs are irritating; even when not irritating, they are harmful, since the body depends more and more upon the drug to do for it what it should be enabled to do for itself, by remedying the original cause of the trouble. Licorice powder, cascara, saline cathartics such as Seidlitz powders and Rochelle Salts and some others are harmless for occasional use, if occasional is not too liberally interpreted.

Tonics are poor substitutes for proper diet, rest, and fresh air. Using them may be likened to beating a tired horse; the horse goes faster, but he is not really stronger. In some emergencies the horse must go faster and there is nothing to do but beat him, and in some cases the tonic should be given; these, however, are cases for a doctor to decide. People persist in taking tonics because they are unwilling or unable to rest, or otherwise to change their ways of living.

Medicines to stop pain or to induce sleep are probably the most pernicious of all self-prescribed remedies, for they add to other dangers the possibility of forming drug habits. These habits are so insidious and so powerful that it is not safe to take habit-forming drugs even once except by a doctor's direction. In short periods of time strong people, apparently firm in will and character, have acquired habits from supposedly moderate use of drugs like morphine, cocaine, and alcohol. No one, no matter how sure of his own self-control, can afford to run so grave a risk.

PATENT REMEDIES.--Objections to self dosing in general apply even more strongly to using patent medicines. The ingredients of patent medicines are ordinarily unknown, so that using them is unintelligent at best. Sometimes they contain habit-forming or other harmful drugs. In other cases the ingredients are innocent enough, but totally unable to bring about the results claimed for them. The old story about a powerful remedy discovered by accident and thus unknown to the medical profession deceives only the ignorant or credulous; with our present knowledge of chemistry and physiology powerful remedies are not discovered in that way.

Even to these comparatively harmless patent preparations there are two serious objections. One is the loss of time, during which the patient may grow worse. The other is that money is obtained under false pretenses; fraud is a common element in the success of patent remedies. One of the least harmful, a substance called "Murine" may be taken as an example[2]. This substance was widely advertised at one time as a "positive cure for sore eyes." Analysis showed it to be a solution of borax, which cost about five cents a gallon to prepare. It sold for one dollar an ounce, or at the rate of $128.00 a gallon. Although it could not bring about the wonderful cures advertised, it was practically harmless, and buyers of "Murine" must have been injured chiefly in pocket. But with "cancer cures" and "consumption cures" it is a different story. Early treatment of these diseases is essential to recovery; delay in many cases means robbing the sufferer of his only chance of life. No drugs are now known that will cure these diseases, and it seems incredible that anyone should be willing to practise such cruel deception upon ignorant people merely for the sake of making money.

ADMINISTRATION OF MEDICINE.--Medicines may be introduced into the body in a number of ways. In the majority of cases they are swallowed and finally carried to the tissues by the blood just as digested food is carried.

Except in rare emergencies no medicine should be given to a sick person without the doctor's order. The prescribed dose should be accurately measured in a medicine glass having a scale to show the number of teaspoonfuls. When measuring medicine, think only of what you are doing; neither talk nor listen to conversation. First read the label on the bottle. Next, shake the bottle, if the medicine is liquid, in order to mix the contents thoroughly. Then remove the cork with the second and third fingers, and hold it between them while pouring, thus keeping the cork clean and protecting the contents of the bottle. Hold the medicine glass on a level with the eyes, and in the other hand hold the bottle, with the side bearing the label uppermost to avoid soiling it; pour out the dose, measuring exactly, wipe the bottle, replace the cork, and again read the label on the bottle.

Most medicines should be diluted with a little water. Pills and capsules should not be presented to patients in the attendant's fingers, but on a saucer or teaspoon. Acids and medicines containing iron should be taken through a glass tube kept for medicine exclusively. Tubes and glasses should be washed at once after use, and neither they nor the bottles should stay in the patient's room. If a dose is omitted for any reason, do not increase the next dose; give the regular dose at the next regular time.

Serious mistakes in giving or taking drugs are far too common, and no precautions are too great to guard against them. Never use medicine from a box or bottle that has no label. Never take or give another person a medicine selected in the dark, even though you have positive knowledge that there is no other bottle or box of medicine in the whole house; in just such circumstances the fatal mistakes occur.

A few things can be done to make medicines more palatable. The water used to dilute the dose and to be taken after it should be very cold. Holding the nose is helpful. A piece of cracker, a peppermint, or a slice of lemon or orange, if allowed, may be taken afterward. Giving disagreeable medicine in ordinary food, as lemon juice, orange juice, or milk, and giving bitter powders in jam or jelly, is unwise because it sometimes results in life long dislike for a useful article of diet. Where food is given directly after the dose to take away its taste, the association of dislike seems to be formed less frequently.

The taste of castor oil is so disgusting that it often causes vomiting, but if skillfully given the oil need not be tasted by a patient who is willing to coöperate. Its way of sticking to the tongue and teeth constitutes the chief difficulty; the object therefore is to prevent it from sticking by swallowing the dose all at once. To administer the oil, wet the inside of a medicine glass or large spoon with very cold water, and leave a little water in the bottom. Pour the required dose in slowly and cover it with more cold water. Let the patient hold in his hand something to take away the taste,--cracker, bread, peppermint, or whatever is allowed; for castor oil water is not very effectual. Then direct him to hold his nose, open his mouth, and hold his breath; caution him to let the oil run down without swallowing until all has been taken, and afterward to chew the cracker, continuing to hold his nose until he has swallowed the cracker. When the patient understands and is ready, pour the dose in quickly as far back as possible, taking care not to spill the last drop on the lips. This process may seem unduly troublesome, but when castor oil is needed it is badly needed and efforts to make it stay down are worth while. The following method also effectually disguises the taste of castor oil: place in a glass a teaspoonful of baking soda, add the prescribed dose of oil and then the juice of half a lemon. Mix all together thoroughly and let the patient take the mixture while it is effervescing. This method may be used unless the patient is not allowed soda and lemon juice. Castor oil may be bought in capsules, but on account of their size many people find the capsules impossible to swallow.

SUPPOSITORIES.--Sometimes medicines are given through the rectum. For this purpose they are combined with cocoa butter or other material, and made into small cones called suppositories. They melt at a low temperature and should be kept on ice until needed. A suppository should be lubricated with vaseline, and inserted very gently as far as the finger can be introduced, while the patient is lying on the back or left side.

ENEMATA.--An injection of a fluid into the rectum is called an enema. (Plural, enemas, or enemata.) Enemas are generally used to cause evacuation of the bowels.

For a simple purgative enema one of the following is generally used: plain water; or a solution of common salt in the proportion of one teaspoonful of salt to one pint of water; or soap suds made with a white soap such as castile or ivory. Unless otherwise ordered the temperature of the enema should be between 105° and 110° F.

To give an enema, one should proceed as follows: First protect the bed by placing under the patient's hips a rubber sheet, covered by a draw sheet or large towel. Let the patient lie on the back, with the knees flexed and head low. Bring to the bedside a commode or bedpan, and lastly the solution contained in a fountain syringe having a long rubber tube, stopcock and short hard rubber nozzle. The bag of the syringe may be hung on the bed post or elsewhere, but it should not be more than three feet at most above the patient's head. Lubricate the nozzle with vaseline either from a tube, or removed from a jar by means of a piece of toilet paper; never dip the nozzle itself into a vaseline jar. Let the solution flow into the bedpan until it runs warm and smoothly; a jerky flow means presence of air bubbles which cause pain if injected into the bowels. Unless the patient is able to do it herself, gently insert the nozzle, and at the same time start the flow. Force must not be used in inserting the nozzle, and the flow should be gentle; if the solution goes in rapidly the patient may be unable to retain it. If there is a desire to expel the enema as soon as the injection has begun, shut off the current and wait a minute, meanwhile making gentle pressure upon the patient's abdomen with one hand; then lower the bag a little and begin again. A grown person should take from two to four pints, and a child from one to two pints. After the enema is finished give the bedpan immediately; the enema will, however, be more effective if retained a few minutes. The bedpan should be given and removed according to the directions on page 176. Sometimes an enema is expelled with such violence that it soils the upper sheet; to protect the covers a rubber sheet may be spread over the patient's knees and legs. Since an enema sometimes causes nausea or faintness, a patient should be watched constantly during the process.

To give an enema to a baby one may use a small syringe having a soft rubber bulb with a nozzle directly attached, or the ordinary fountain syringe with the small, hard rubber tip designed for infants. The enema should be given in a warm room free from draughts, and the baby must be warmly covered throughout the process. First cover the lap with a pad or folded blanket. Upon the blanket place a warmed rubber sheet, and over the rubber a warm diaper. Hold the baby on your lap, so that he lies on his back with his knees drawn up. Hold his feet or legs firmly in your left hand. Lubricate the nozzle thoroughly with vaseline. Be sure that all the air is expelled from the syringe, and then proceed as already directed. A baby will take from two or three ounces up to half a pint or even more, according to the size of the child. After the injection is finished place a small vessel under the baby's hips, and hold it until the fluid has been expelled, keeping the child well covered all the time.

After being used, the nozzle of a fountain syringe should be washed with soap and water, boiled, dried and put away in a clean place. Inserting the nozzle into the bag of the syringe immediately after withdrawing it from the rectum is a filthy but not uncommon practice. The syringe should be kept clean inside and out; it should be washed in hot soapsuds, rinsed in clean hot water, drained, and when thoroughly dry wrapped in a clean towel or tissue paper. The ordinary fountain syringe hanging for months by a dirty string on a hook in the bath room is an unpleasant and generally an unclean object.

SPRAYS AND GARGLES.--Several other methods of administering medicines are occasionally employed. Some remedies may be applied directly to the throat by gargles, and to the nose and throat by sprays. The throat may be cleansed by gargling with a solution of a teaspoonful of baking soda or common salt in a glass of warm water. Nose sprays should not be used except under medical advice, and it is well to remember that if the mouth washes, gargles, and sprays advertised to be disinfectants were really strong enough to kill germs, they would be too harsh for common or continued use. The nozzles of nose and throat sprays should be boiled immediately after use. A surprising number of families who have progressed far beyond common drinking cups and towels, continue to use a common nose spray without even washing the nozzle. Children while they are well should be taught to gargle the throat; a child with a sore throat and an aching head is in a poor condition to learn anything.

INHALATION or breathing in, is another method used to introduce drugs into the membranes of the nose, throat, and lungs. Smelling salts are an example of substances used for inhalation; they are used to stimulate persons who are faint. They should not be placed close to the nostrils, nor used at all when the patient is totally unconscious.

Inhalations of steam are often used in asthma, croup, and bronchitis. Special croup kettles are made for the purpose, but an ordinary pitcher half full of boiling water may be used instead. The patient's head should be held closely over the pitcher, and a towel should be adjusted around the top covering the patient's nose and mouth, but admitting just enough air to make it possible for him to breathe. If a drug is ordered it should be added to the water.

INUNCTION, or rubbing a substance into the skin, is sometimes ordered for delicate babies and children. After the skin of the abdomen has been washed with warm soapy water and thoroughly dried, the substance ordered, generally olive oil or cod liver oil, should be applied by means of a circular movement of the palm of the hand. The oil should be warm and the rubbing continued until it is absorbed.

Ointments are also applied by inunction. A small quantity at a time should be rubbed in, using a circular motion. If an ointment is ordered to be applied where the skin is broken, the ointment should be spread upon gauze and applied without friction. Liniments are rubbed in in the same way as ointments. In many cases rubbing accomplishes more than the ointment or liniment itself, so that this part of the treatment must not be slighted.

HOUSEHOLD MEDICINE CUPBOARD.--In every household a small cupboard is needed for medical and surgical supplies. Glass shelves are desirable, because they show when dirty and are easily cleaned, but a wooden cupboard can easily be lined with clean paper or white enamel cloth held in place with thumb tacks. Dirty, stained shelves should not be tolerated. The cupboard should be kept locked and the key put well out of the reach of children. In the cupboard should be kept medicines in daily use; they should not be paraded on family dinner tables.

Poisonous drugs should have rough glass bottles and conspicuous labels. All medicine bottles should be kept well corked, since evaporation may take place and the remaining solution, by becoming stronger, may be dangerous to use in the ordinary amount. Pills and tablets sometimes deteriorate by standing, and may become so hard that they pass through the stomach and intestines without dissolving. It is best to buy drugs and surgical supplies in small quantities; when it is cheaper to buy more at a time the druggist should be asked whether they will deteriorate or not.

Almost every family needs to keep on hand some cathartics, some disinfectants, some material for first aid, and a few simple appliances. Most families have certain other needs peculiar to themselves, and for those who live at a distance from drug stores a greater quantity and variety may be required. Elaborate equipment and extensive supplies of medicines are neither economical nor necessary for household use.

Castor oil, Rochelle or other laxative salts, and two grain cascara tablets ordinarily constitute a sufficient supply of cathartics. The dose of castor oil is one or two teaspoonfuls for a baby up to a tablespoonful for an adult. Rochelle salts and seltzer aperient are given dissolved in water; the ordinary dose is from one to four teaspoonfuls. Seidlitz powders come in two packets, one white and one blue. The contents of the packets should first be dissolved in separate glasses each filled about a quarter full of water. One solution should then be poured into the other and the mixture taken while it is effervescing. Cascara tablets are generally given in one to ten grain doses.

A small bottle of tincture of iodine and one of 70% alcohol should be kept for disinfecting. Neither one is for internal use. The iodine is used to disinfect small wounds and abrasions of the skin. It is applied with cotton swabs and several swabs should be made and kept on hand in a box or envelope. Alcohol is used to disinfect thermometers and other instruments that cannot be boiled, for rubbing, and may also be used for disinfecting the skin. A 90% solution is sometimes used for rubbing; it need not be bought until needed. Denatured and wood alcohol are poisons and should be used in households only in spirit lamps; they are not safe for other purposes.

First aid materials may include two gauze bandages two and one-half inches wide and two bandages one inch wide, one American Red Cross First Aid Outfit, a small package of absorbent cotton, a roll of old muslin, a package of adhesive plaster one inch wide, boracic ointment, picric acid gauze or other application for burns, safety pins, and a pair of scissors.

For use in cases of fainting or exhaustion it is well to keep aromatic spirits of ammonia on hand. Its bottle should have a rubber stopper. The dose is one-half to one teaspoonful, in a quarter to half a glass of water. Hot coffee and tea are also good stimulants, but the time necessary to prepare them makes it desirable to have aromatic ammonia on hand. Household or ordinary ammonia must not be used as a substitute.

Olive oil, mustard, and baking soda may be brought from the kitchen when needed. It is assumed that vaseline, cold cream, hand lotion, talcum powder, and other toilet preparations will also be available.

Only a few appliances are necessary. Among them are a medicine glass, a teaspoon, clinical thermometer, hot water bag, fountain syringe, and an alcohol lamp in houses without gas or electric stoves. It is better not to buy other appliances until they are needed, particularly rubber goods since they deteriorate rapidly.

EXERCISES

1. Why is it dangerous for persons without medical training to prescribe medicines? What is the especial danger of dosing oneself?

2. What is meant by a habit-forming drug? Name all you can, and tell why they are peculiarly dangerous.

3. What are the special objections to patent medicines?

4. What precautions should be taken in order to administer medicine accurately? What precautions to avoid giving wrong medicines?

5. How may some disagreeable medicines be made more palatable?

6. Tell how to prepare and give a soapsuds enema.

7. How should a fountain syringe be cared for? a throat spray?

8. Describe methods for giving steam inhalations.

9. Describe the equipment and care of a household medicine cupboard.

10. What drugs is it well for a family to keep on hand? What appliances? What materials for first aid?

11. How many drugs in addition to those prescribed by a physician have you or your family on hand at the present time? How many do you consider really necessary? Are any of these medicines used to remedy troubles that might be cured by sufficient attention to rest, exercise, diet, and fresh air?

FOR FURTHER READING

Health and Disease--Roger I. Lee, Chapter VI.

How to Live--Fisher and Fisk, Supplementary Notes, Sections IV, V.

Scientific Features of Modern Medicine--Frederic S. Lee, Chapters III, VIII.

The Human Mechanism--Hough and Sedgwick, Chapter XX.

The Conquest of Nerves--Courtney.

Primitive Psychotherapy and Quackery--Lawrence, Chapters I-V.

Nostrums and Quackery--American Medical Association. (See especially "Cancer Cures" and "Consumption Cures.")

FOOTNOTES:

[2] See "Nostrums and Quackery," p. 445.

CHAPTER XI

APPLICATION OF HEAT, COLD, AND COUNTER-IRRITANTS

INFLAMMATION.--A process called inflammation sometimes occurs in tissues that have been injured or invaded by bacteria. Although painful, it is nevertheless one of the reparative processes of the body, and therefore beneficial. Common examples of inflammation are boils, sore throat, and the swollen, painful condition resulting from sprains and fractures. Characteristic symptoms of inflammation are heat, redness, swelling, and pain.

When a tissue has been invaded by bacteria, nearby blood vessels dilate, thus bringing an increased supply of blood to the affected part. This extra supply serves to wash away the offending substance, and at the same time it brings more white blood corpuscles, one function of which is to destroy bacteria. From the increased supply of blood the affected part becomes red and hot, and so much blood may come that the vessels further on are unable to carry it away fast enough. Some of the fluid part of the blood is then forced out into the tissues, and the part becomes swollen. Distension of the tissues and pressure on the nerve endings cause pain, and the injured part now exhibits the characteristic symptoms of inflammation.

[Illustration: FIG. 21.--"THE HISTORY OF A BOIL." This figure represents a cross-section of normal skin. Note the surface layer, or cuticle, and the "true skin," or cutis. In the cutis one sees that the blood capillaries are just wide enough for the blood-cells to pass through "in single file." The skin has just been pricked by a dirty pin. On the point of this pin were several poisonous germs which were deposited at *a*. (*From Emerson's "Essentials of Medicine."*)]

[Illustration: FIG. 22.--"THE HISTORY OF A BOIL" (continued). The poison from these germs diffuses through the cutis. The capillaries dilate. The leucocytes force their way through the walls of the capillaries and travel towards these germs. Note the dumb-bell shape of the leucocytes as they pass through the minute holes in the capillary walls, and their pseudopods as they travel towards their common destination, attracted by the poison from the germs. The skin in this region is now swollen, red, hot, and painful. (*From Emerson's "Essentials of Medicine."*)]

At this point, if the injury begins to heal or the bacterial infection to yield, the extra blood supply is gradually carried off, the blood vessels resume their normal size, and the tissues return to their usual condition. If, however, the infection does not yield so quickly, more and more white blood corpuscles assemble and pass through the walls of the tiny blood vessels into the tissues. Here the struggle continues. Some bacteria and some white blood corpuscles are killed, and substances are formed which liquify these dead cells and also some cells of the surrounding tissues. The resulting fluid is called pus or matter, and in the case of a boil we then say it has come to a head. If the infection occurs near a cavity or near the surface of the body, the pus may escape by breaking through at the point of least resistance, and may carry most of the poisons along with it. If the pus finds no outlet it may be gradually absorbed by the blood stream, and healing may result without discharging. On the other hand, the germs may make their way into the circulation, thus causing the serious condition known as blood poisoning.

[Illustration: FIG. 23.--"THE HISTORY OF A BOIL" (continued). The migration of leucocytes has continued until now they form a dense mass surrounding the germs. The poison of the germs has killed all the leucocytes and also all the cutis immediately around them, and now digestive fluids from the dead leucocytes is turning the whole dead mass into liquid pus. The boil has "come to a head." There is a little lump on the skin and through its thin covering of cuticle can be seen the yellow pus. (*From Emerson's "Essentials of Medicine."*)]

Inflammation may be treated by means of hot applications, cold applications, or counter-irritants. The effect of heat is to dilate the vessels and hence to increase the flow of blood to the injured part. This increased blood supply makes the reparative process go on more vigorously, and also makes it possible for the accumulated fluid to be more rapidly carried away. Moist heat softens the tissues so that pus, if formed, can escape more easily.

[Illustration: FIG. 24.--"THE HISTORY OF A BOIL" (concluded). The boil has finally ruptured. The liquid pus has escaped carrying with it the germs and most of their poisons; the migration of leucocytes has stopped; the capillaries are returning to normal size and now new tissue will grow and fill up this hole. (*From Emerson's "Essentials of Medicine."*)]

Cold acts in just the opposite way. It decreases the size of the blood vessels so that less blood comes to cause pain and swelling; at the same time it diminishes the number of white blood corpuscles and the nutritive substance brought by the blood. The nature and location of the infection determine whether heat or cold is to be preferred.

Counter-irritants, of which mustard is an example, have a complicated action. A counter-irritant affects the blood circulation of the place to which it is applied, and at the same time it irritates the superficial nerves, which in turn stimulate other more distant nerves. The latter nerves control the circulation in tissues not adjoining those to which the counter-irritant is applied, and thus it is possible for a mustard paste, for example, if applied at one point to bring about changes in the blood supply of another part of the body. The mechanism by which counter-irritation is brought about is an intricate nervous process called reflex action.

HOT APPLICATIONS

In applying either moist or dry heat the danger of burning or scalding a patient must be constantly kept in mind. This danger is always great, but it is especially great when the skin is tender like that of babies, children, and old people, or when the vitality is low as in cases of chronic or exhausting illness. Unfortunately accidents in applying heat are not uncommon; a moment's carelessness may cause serious injury and prolonged suffering.

DRY HEAT.--Hot water bags are used to apply dry heat. They should be filled not more than two-thirds full of hot water, but the water must not be so hot that there is the slightest possibility of scalding the patient if the bag should leak. Boiling water should never be used. Before the stopper is screwed on, expel the air by squeezing the bag or by resting it upon a flat surface until the water reaches the top. After closing the bag make sure that both bag and stopper are in order, by noting whether leakage occurs when the bag is inverted and pressed moderately. Before it is placed near the patient the bag should be dried and entirely covered with a towel or canton flannel bag.

Strong bottles, jugs, and jars, if they can be securely stoppered, may be used sometimes instead of hot water bags. The same precautions are necessary. Bricks, flat irons, or thick flannel bags containing salt or sand may be heated in the oven and used in the same way. Salt and sand retain heat for a long time, but are correspondingly slow to heat; therefore one bag should be heating in the oven while the other is in use. Their effect on the skin must be no less carefully watched than the effects of other hot applications.

Hot dry flannel may be used without fear of burning a patient, and it sometimes yields sufficient warmth to relieve pain, particularly abdominal pain of babies. After it has been heated on a radiator or in an oven, it should be applied quickly and covered closely with another flannel to prevent escape of heat.

Dry heat can be applied conveniently by an electric pad. The part to be heated may be wrapped in flannel or placed directly above or below the pad. The pad should be carefully watched to see that the switch is not accidentally turned, as it is possible for the pad to become hot enough to burn the patient or to set fire to the bed covers.

MOIST HEAT.--To apply moist heat poultices or fomentations (stupes) are used.

Poultices may be made of various heat-retaining substances, but flaxseed meal is generally used. The poultices when ready should be applied without delay, therefore all preparations should be made in advance. To prepare a poultice, first provide a piece of gauze or thin old muslin about two inches wider than you wish the poultice to be when finished, and about two inches more than twice as long. In a shallow saucepan boil water, varying in amount according to the size of the poultice desired; about equal parts of water and meal will be needed. When the water is boiling briskly add the meal gradually, beating constantly with a spatula or knife. The poultice is done when the mixture coheres and is thick enough to drop from the spatula leaving it clean. Quickly spread a layer of the hot flaxseed from a quarter to half an inch thick on one-half of the muslin, leaving a margin on three sides of about an inch (Fig. 25). Fold in the margins of the cloth (Fig. 26) and then bring the other half of the cloth over the flaxseed so that the top of the poultice is covered. Tuck the free end of the upper half of the cloth under the turned in edges of the long sides.

[Illustration: FIG. 25.--Turn the edges of the muslin over the flaxseed by folding first on the line *AA'*, and then on the lines *BB'* and *CC'*.]

[Illustration: FIG. 26.--Fold on the line *EE'*, bringing *FF'* up over the flaxseed and tucking it under at *D* and *D'*.]

Carry the poultice on a hot plate, or rolled in a newspaper or hot towel. Test it carefully with the back of the hand, apply it to the skin gradually, cover it with cotton batting, oiled muslin, or several thicknesses of flannel, and keep it in place with a bandage or towel. Remove it as soon as it has become cold, and unless the skin is much reddened apply a fresh poultice. If the skin is much reddened, anoint it with vaseline or sweet oil, wrap it warmly, and apply the next poultice as soon as the appearance of the skin is normal.

Stupes or *hot fomentations* are cloths, preferably of flannel or flannelette, wrung out of boiling water and applied to the skin. Each stupe should be three or four times as large as the area to be covered. Two are needed, so that one may be prepared before removing the other. To prevent escape of heat and moisture the stupe should be covered after it has been applied, first with a piece of rubber cloth or oiled silk or muslin, and next with several thicknesses of flannel, or cotton batting made into a pad. The whole should be kept in place with a bandage or towel used as a binder. The doctor will tell how often the stupes are to be applied, but if the skin becomes irritated they must be stopped until its appearance is again normal.

[Illustration: FIG. 27.--WRINGING STUPE. (*From "Elementary Nursing Procedures," California State Board of Health.*)]

Great care must be taken in applying fomentations. They do little good unless very hot, but if applied too hot the patient is likely to be scalded. They must be wrung as dry as possible; but it is difficult to wring them without scalding the hands unless stupe wringers are used. Stupe wringers are heavy pieces of cloth, like roller towels or pieces of ticking, long enough to extend over opposite sides of the basin in which the stupe is to be boiled, and wide enough to hold the stupe easily. The wringer should be placed in the basin with the stupe arranged upon it. Boiling water should then be added, or the water, stupe, and wringer may be boiled together in the basin. After the stupe is ready, the wringer with the stupe upon it should be removed from the water by grasping the dry ends of the wringer. Then the ends should be twisted in opposite directions until the stupe inside is as dry as possible. Wringing is made easier if the wringer has wide hems into which sticks such as pieces of broom handles are inserted. By twisting the sticks in opposite directions the stupe may be wrung out easily.

COLD APPLICATIONS

DRY COLD.--Cold, like heat, may be used either dry or moist. Bags of rubber or of Japanese paper filled with small pieces of ice are used to apply dry cold. When weight is to be avoided, the bag should not be completely filled. After the bag has been filled and the air has been expelled, it should be stoppered securely and wrapped in a towel or piece of flannel, since it is possible for an uncovered ice bag to freeze the skin. Ice bags are easily punctured, and care should be taken not to bring pressure upon them especially when filled with sharp pieces of ice. An ice bag not in use should be thoroughly dry inside and out; it should be put away with enough absorbent cotton inside to keep the surfaces from adhering. Bags of Japanese paper are less costly than rubber, but less durable. To close them one should roll the top over and then tie it tightly with string.

MOIST COLD.--Cold compresses for the head are often used for patients with fever or headache; they sometimes quiet a patient who is restless. An old handkerchief or piece of soft linen folded with the raw edges inside may be used as a compress. It should be large enough to cover the forehead. Two compresses at least should be provided, and a large piece of ice in a basin. One compress should be wrung so that it will not drip, and then applied to the head. The other meanwhile should be placed on the ice to cool. As soon as the first compress becomes warm, the second should be applied in its place.

Cold Compresses for the Eyes.--Soft material should be selected for eye compresses. Each one should be cut only a little larger than the eye and should fit neatly over it. Several compresses should be placed on a block of ice while one is applied to the eye, and every few minutes the compress should be changed. If there is discharge from the eye, each compress should be used but once; when used, they should be collected in a paper and afterward burned. Separate compresses should be used if both eyes are being treated. Definite directions in regard to changing compresses and the length of time the applications should be continued are generally given by the physician.

COUNTER-IRRITANTS

To some extent all hot applications are counter-irritants, but mustard pastes, mustard leaves, and the mustard foot-bath already described are the counter-irritants most commonly used.

Mustard Paste.--To make a mustard paste, mix dry mustard with flour, using for adults one part of mustard and six of flour to make a weak paste; increase the proportion of mustard up to equal parts of mustard and flour, according to the strength required. Use a smaller proportion of mustard for children; one part of mustard with from 6 to 10 parts of flour is generally enough. Add to the mustard and flour enough tepid water to make a paste, which must be absolutely free from lumps. Do not use hot water for this purpose, because it destroys some of the active properties of the mustard. Spread the paste on thin muslin, apply it to the skin, and remove it as soon as the skin is reddened so that its color resembles that of a strong sun-burn. If the skin is especially sensitive, mix a little sweet oil or vaseline with the paste.

Mustard leaves should be dipped in tepid water and may then be applied to the skin directly, but if specially sensitive, the skin should be protected by thin muslin or gauze. The leaf should remain until the skin is well reddened; a few minutes are generally sufficient.

Care must be taken not to leave either a mustard leaf or a paste in place long enough to blister the skin. After the application has been removed; the part should be protected by a soft cloth until redness disappears. Vaseline or sweet oil should be applied to the skin if it is greatly irritated.

Other counter-irritants in common use are iodine, turpentine, ammonia, kerosene, camphorated oil, capsicum vaseline, and various liniments. Tincture of iodine may be diluted with alcohol for especially sensitive skins; it sometimes causes blisters, and should not be applied more than once a day at most. Ammonia and turpentine cause blisters; they should not be used as counter-irritants except by a doctor's order, and then only after exact directions have been obtained. Turpentine and kerosene are inflammable and hence dangerous to use. It should be remembered that the action of all counter-irritants is physiologically the same, so that no advantage is obtained from the use of dangerous substances like kerosene and turpentine.

EXERCISES

1. What are the causes and symptoms of inflammation?

2. Describe the process of inflammation.

3. What is the effect of heat on an inflamed area? of cold?

4. What are the dangers from hot applications, and how may they be guarded against?

5. How should you fill a hot water bag? How should you cover it?

6. Describe the method of preparing and applying a flaxseed poultice.

7. Tell how to prepare and apply fomentations.

8. How should you apply cold compresses to the head? to the eyes?

9. How should you make a mustard paste for a baby six months old? for a grown person only slightly ill? for a feeble old person with a

sensitive skin?

FOR FURTHER READING

Essentials of Medicine--Emerson, Chapter I.

The Human Mechanism--Hough and Sedgwick, Chapter IX.

CHAPTER XII

CARE OF PATIENTS WITH COMMUNICABLE DISEASES

The first chapter of this book described the ways in which communicable diseases are carried from person to person, and also some principles underlying methods of prevention. This chapter aims to show how these principles apply in the actual care of patients whose diseases are transmissible. In order to apply them intelligently, it is necessary to keep in mind certain facts in regard to the transmission of infections. A brief summary of these facts follows.

Disease germs are present in the bodies of persons suffering from communicable disease, but they may also exist in the bodies of persons in good health; if present in the body, they may leave it in any bodily discharge. While every kind of germ does not leave the body by all the different routes, it is nevertheless true that most germs expelled from the body are carried in discharges from the nose, throat, bladder or bowels. Germ-laden discharges of an infected person may be distributed to other persons by water, milk and other foods, by certain insects, by unclean hands, by common drinking cups, towels, handkerchiefs, and similar articles, and directly by nose and throat spray. After they have been thus conveyed to other persons, the germs make their entrance into the body of their new victims through the digestive tract, through the nose, throat, and other mucous membranes, or through breaks in the skin. Prevention of communicable diseases, therefore, depends upon the measure of success attained in blocking the transit of germs from person to person; but methods of prevention, though easy to understand, are unfortunately sometimes difficult to carry out. In order to carry them out effectively one must devote to the problem great accuracy, unremitting care, considerable intelligence, and a highly developed conscience.

Care of a patient suffering from transmissible disease is adequate only when it accomplishes two definite results. One result, which concerns the patient primarily, is to bring about his recovery as rapidly and as surely as possible; the other result, which concerns the community rather than the individual, is to make it impossible for the patient to infect others with his disease. In every case of communicable disease, from a slight cold in the head up to serious cases of pneumonia or typhoid fever, both the patient and the community must be constantly safe-guarded.

INCUBATION PERIOD.--The interval between the moment when pathogenic germs enter the body, and the time when symptoms first appear and the patient begins to feel ill, is called the incubation period. Incubation periods vary according to the disease from a few hours to two or three weeks. The length of the period also varies somewhat in different cases of the same disease.

CARE OF PATIENTS WITH COLDS OR OTHER SLIGHT INFECTIONS.--The usual symptoms of infectious diseases include fever, chill, sore throat, nasal discharge, cough, headache, vomiting and other digestive disturbances, and a general feeling of being sick all over. When one or more of these symptoms appear, unless they are very slight, a doctor should be sent for. The patient, whether child or grown person, should go to bed in a room alone and should stay in bed at least as long as the fever and symptoms of cold in the head continue, in order to protect others as well as himself. Persons in active life, it is true, are not always able to go to bed during colds; but there is no doubt that ultimately they would save time by doing so. It is especially necessary for children to remain in bed when suffering from colds, not only to insure their own well-being but also to protect others, since children are notably careless in regard to coughing, sneezing, and borrowing handkerchiefs. The patient needs mental rest as well as physical, and should not be allowed to work in bed.

The patient's nose and throat discharges should be received only in material that can be burned, like old linen or muslin, gauze, or paper napkins. As soon as they are soiled these handkerchief substitutes should be placed in strong paper bags and afterward burned. Soiled handkerchiefs lurking under pillows or in other parts of the bed may infect other people or re-infect the patient. Handkerchiefs that may not be burned should be placed as soon as soiled in a covered receptacle filled with cold water containing a little washing soda; when several have been collected they should be boiled in the same covered receptacle for 20 minutes. After boiling they may go to the regular laundry.

The patient's diet at first should be liquid or semi-solid. Large amounts of nourishment are not necessary during the first day or two, especially if the illness is likely to be short, but water should be taken as freely as possible. Cold drinks are generally acceptable during the feverish stage, but lemonade and other acids should be used with caution, since they sometimes irritate a sore throat. When the active symptoms have subsided the patient will need more food than usual, and a liberal, nourishing diet for a few days will do much to prevent the weakness and depressed vitality that often follow colds, tonsilitis, and other comparatively slight infections.

The bowels should be carefully regulated, and a mild cathartic is often beneficial at the outset.

Even during slight illness a patient should receive the daily care already described, and should be made as comfortable as possible. As in any illness, sponging and alcohol rubs are refreshing. An ice bag or cold compress may relieve headache, and hot applications or a cold compress on the throat are often soothing. The throat may be gargled with a solution of one teaspoonful of common salt dissolved in a pint of boiled water. If the patient perspires profusely he should be rubbed with a towel until dry, and provided with fresh warm, night clothes. An alcohol rub may well follow. It is most unwise for a patient who is perspiring freely to get up in a cold room and attend to himself.

Common colds are far more serious than they are usually supposed to be.

"More people suffer from common colds than from any other single ailment.... Could the sum total of suffering, inconvenience, sequelæ, and economic loss resulting from common colds be obtained, it would at once promote these infections from the trivial into the rank of the serious diseases.... Colds are contracted from other persons having colds, just as diphtheria is contracted from diphtheria. Arctic explorers exposed to all the conditions ordinarily supposed to produce colds do not suffer from these ailments until they return to civilization and become infected by contact with their fellowmen.... While common colds are never fatal, the complications and sequelæ are serious. These are rheumatic fever, pneumonia, sinusitis, nephritis, and a depressed vitality which favors other infections and hastens the progress of organic diseases.

"Common colds are perhaps most contagious during the early stages. If persons isolate themselves by remaining in bed during the first three days of a cold, they would not only benefit themselves, but would largely prevent the spread of the infection. The contagiousness and severity of colds differ in different epidemics and in different seasons of the year, depending upon the particular micro-organism involved and other factors not well understood.

"PREVENTION.--The prevention of colds consists, first in avoiding the infection, and, secondly, in guarding against the predisposing causes. Contact should be avoided with persons who have colds, especially in street cars, offices, and other poorly ventilated spaces where the risk of persons coughing or sneezing directly in one's face is imminent. Contact with the infection may further be guarded against by a careful self-education in sanitary habits and cleanliness, based upon the modern conception of contact infection.

"Colds, like other diseases conveyed in the secretions from the nose and mouth, are often conveyed by direct and indirect contact through lack of hygienic cleanliness and a disregard of sanitary habits. Kissing, the common drinking cup, the roller towel, pipes, toys, pencils, fingers, food, and other objects contaminated with the fresh secretions will transmit the disease."--("Preventive Medicine and Hygiene," Rosenau.)

CARE DURING MORE SERIOUS INFECTIONS.--When a patient is suffering from serious transmissible disease, he needs the most skillful care available, and for the sake of others he must be strictly isolated or quarantined. By isolating or quarantining a patient is meant making such arrangements that germs expelled by the patient are necessarily destroyed before they can enter the body of another person. Isolation, therefore, includes disinfection, and while methods vary according to the nature of the particular disease, yet the principles given below are applicable in most cases.

The first essential is that the patient should have a room to himself. No one except those caring for him should enter the sick-room for any purpose whatever; visitors should be rigidly excluded. At the outset all unnecessary articles should be removed from the sick-room, and it should be possible to boil, burn, scrub, or otherwise thoroughly clean everything allowed to remain. The windows should be screened in summer, and flies must be excluded. Fresh air is especially needed by patients with communicable diseases, and ventilation of the room must be adequate both day and night. Foul odors plainly indicate that the patient or something in the room is not clean. The remedy is obvious and deodorants are quite unnecessary if the patient and the room are properly cared for. It is highly desirable to reserve a bath room for the exclusive use of the patient and his attendant and also to reserve a room adjoining the patient's room for the exclusive use of the attendant. When it is impossible, as it often is, to give up so much space, each family must make the best arrangement it can to separate the patient and his attendant from the rest of the family.

The attendant must remember that her ten fingers are the ten most active agents in distributing the communicable diseases. After handling the patient or anything that the patient has touched, and whenever she leaves the patient's room, she must scrub her hands thoroughly with warm water, soap, and a nail brush. She should not soil her hands unnecessarily, even though she intends to scrub them later. She must remember for her own protection to keep her hands away from her mouth and face, and to cleanse them with special care just before eating. If disinfection is needed in addition to the scrubbing, she must use conscientiously whatever solution the doctor orders.

At the same time that she is caring for a patient with a communicable disease, the attendant ought not to care for children or other members of the family, she ought not to prepare food, and she ought not to handle dishes or utensils used by other persons. Every day, however, many women are doing just these things, and it is true that in many instances no bad results are observed. Yet if any arrangement to insure safety can possibly be made, it is inexcusable to run the risk of spreading diseases which kill thousands of persons every year and injure many more for life.

When home conditions render adequate care and strict isolation of the patient impossible, hospital care should be seriously considered. No personal or sentimental objections should be allowed to influence the decision, if removing the patient to a hospital is necessary to safeguard his welfare or the welfare of the family. Hospital care should be considered especially for patients with typhoid fever, because untrained persons cannot safely care for patients so seriously ill. Since a patient with typhoid needs skilled care, and since he greatly endangers other persons, most authorities consider hospital care essential unless the patient can have the continuous services of a trained nurse and almost ideal home conditions. Many cases of typhoid, it is true, are successfully nursed at home in extremely adverse conditions by visiting nurses; yet in few kinds of sickness is continuous care by a graduate nurse more necessary to protect the community as well as to safeguard the patient himself.

Members of a family in which there is typhoid should be immunized if the doctor advises it. This process, which is performed by the doctor, in the majority of cases renders a person immune to typhoid fever for three or four years.

The question of home or institutional care for persons with tuberculosis must also be carefully considered. In some cases tuberculosis may be cared for at home with comparative safety, and in some other cases the risk is not very great if the patient is intelligent, careful, and well supervised. But everyone should face the fact that all cases of tuberculosis of the lungs involve some risk to others in the family, and most cases involve great risk. The danger to children is greater than to adults. Most tuberculosis infections, it is now believed, are acquired in childhood. The bad results of an infection acquired in childhood may not show themselves for years, since the germs may remain inactive until the person's resistance is lowered by some unfavorable condition.

THE CHILDREN'S DISEASES.--The so-called children's diseases are probably the most familiar and the least regarded of all those belonging to the communicable group. Most persons, it is true, realize that scarlet fever is serious; everyone should also realize that measles and whooping-cough are serious. For example, in the State of New York during the year 1916, more children died from each of these diseases than from scarlet fever: in that year 745, or four times the number that died of scarlet fever, lost their lives from whooping-cough, while 913 died of measles. If diseases that kill hundreds of children every year are not serious, one is at a loss to know what a serious disease is.

Some parents even expose children unnecessarily to these infections on the fatalistic theory that they must have the diseases sometime, and therefore the sooner the better. Nothing could be more mistaken; the diseases are not inevitable, and there is no advantage whatever in having them if escape is possible. Moreover, serious as the children's diseases are in themselves, their after-effects may be even more serious. At this very moment hundreds of people are going through life handicapped by weakened hearts or kidneys, by defective sight or hearing, merely because their parents considered the children's diseases necessary. The common belief that children should have these diseases as early as possible is also erroneous, since statistics show that the younger the child the more likely is the disease to prove fatal.

Every mother should realize that the children's diseases are most infectious in the early stages. Early symptoms include fever, sore throat, and nasal discharge, and the trouble at first often resembles a severe cold. During this stage the diseases are most easily communicated. Measles in particular is generally not recognized until its most infectious stage has passed. The moral to be drawn is that sore throats, coughs, and colds should never be regarded lightly, and that their spread should be prevented by all possible means.

The accompanying table taken from the regulations of the New York State Department of Health, gives symptoms of communicable diseases among children, and rules for isolation and exclusion from school.

NEW YORK STATE DEPARTMENT OF HEALTH COMMUNICABLE DISEASES AMONG CHILDREN RULES FOR ISOLATION AND EXCLUSION FROM SCHOOL

HERMAN M. BIGGS, M.D. Commissioner

Issued by the Division of Public Health Education

===

DISEASE | PRINCIPAL SIGNS | METHOD OF | | AND SYMPTOMS |
INFECTION | --------------+------------------------------+----------------------+
CHICKENPOX | Rarely begins with fever. | Contact with discharges | |
Rash appears on second day | from nose and throat of | | as small
pimples, which in | a patient. | | about a day become filled | | | with clear
fluid. This fluid | | | becomes yellow colored, a | | | crust forms and the
scab | | | falls off in about 14 days. | | | Successive crops of papules | | |
appear until tenth day. | |
--------------+------------------------------+----------------------+ DIPHTHERIA |
Onset may be rapid or | Contact with discharges | | gradual. The back
of the | from nose and throat, | | throat, tonsils, or palate | occasionally
by | | may show patches. The most | drinking infected milk. | |
pronounced symptom is sore | | | throat. There may be hardly | | | any
symptoms at all. | |
--------------+------------------------------+----------------------+ MEASLES |
Begins like cold in the | Contact with discharges | | head, with running
nose, | from nose and throat | | sneezing, inflamed and | of a patient. | |
watery eyes and fever. | | | Mulberry-tinted spots appear | | | about the
third day; rash | | | first seen behind the ears, | | | on forehead and face.
The | | | rash varies with heat; may | | | almost disappear if the air | | | is
cold, and come out again, | | | with warmth. | |
--------------+------------------------------+----------------------+ MEASLES |
Illness usually slight. | Same as above. | (LIBERTY) | Onset sudden.
Lymph nodes in | | | back of neck enlarged. Rash | | | often first thing
noticed; | | | no cold in head. Usually | | | have fever, sore throat, and | |
| the eyes may be inflamed. | | | Rash sometimes resembles | | |
measles and scarlet fever, | | | variable. | |
--------------+------------------------------+----------------------+ MUMPS |
Onset may be sudden, | Same as above. | | beginning with sickness
and | | | fever, and pain about the | | | angle of the jaw. The | | | parotid
glands become | | | swollen and tender. Opening | | | the mouth is
accompanied by | | | pain. | |
--------------+------------------------------+----------------------+
POLIOMYELITIS| Onset sudden, fever, | Contact with discharge | |
excitable, pain on bending | from nose, throat or | | neck forward, pain
on being | bowels of a patient | | handled, headache, vomiting. | or
carrier. | | Sometimes sudden development | | | of weakness of one or
more | | | muscle groups. | |

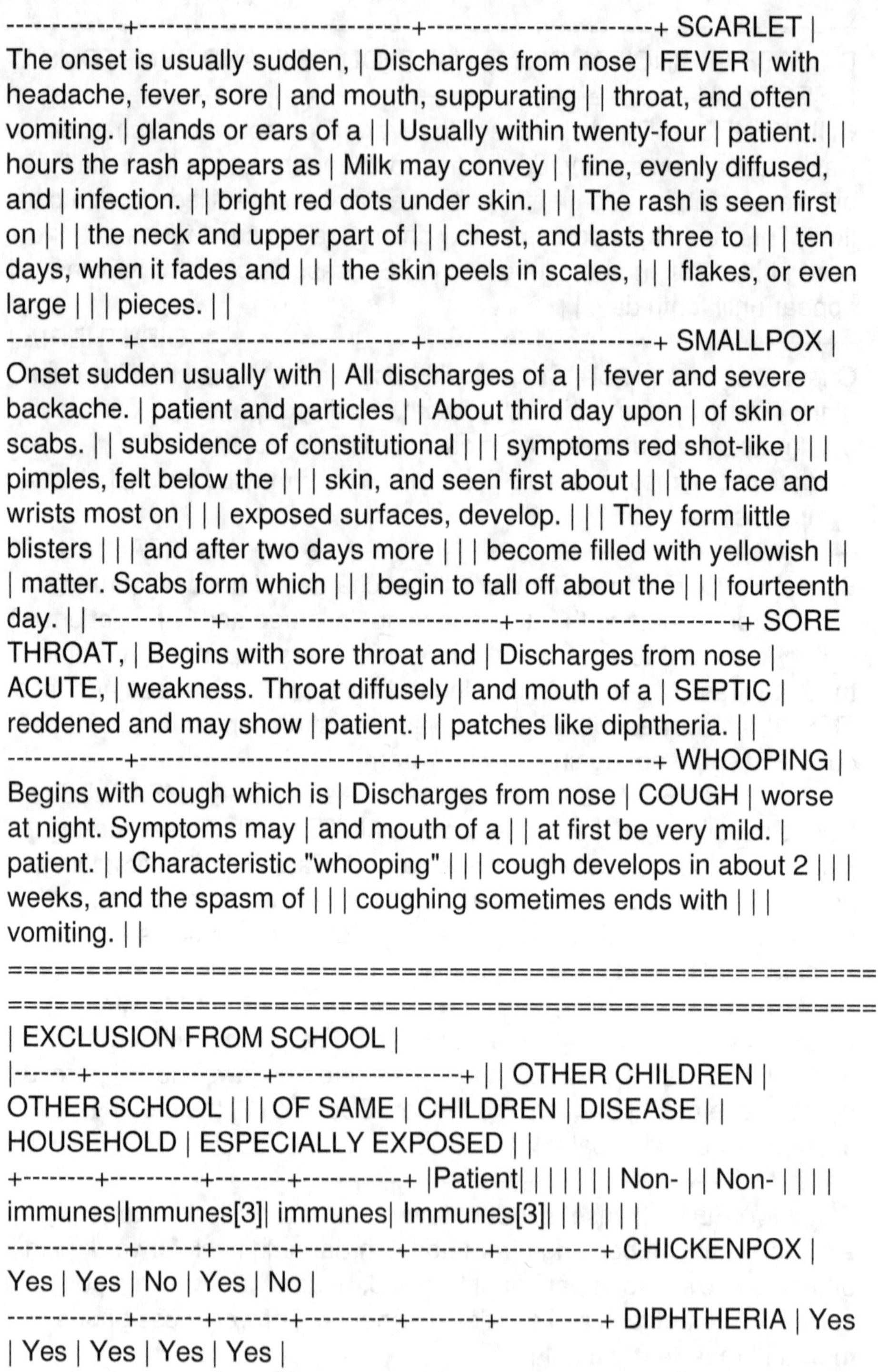

-------------+----------------------------+-----------------------+ SCARLET |
The onset is usually sudden, | Discharges from nose | FEVER | with
headache, fever, sore | and mouth, suppurating | | throat, and often
vomiting. | glands or ears of a | | Usually within twenty-four | patient. | |
hours the rash appears as | Milk may convey | | fine, evenly diffused,
and | infection. | | bright red dots under skin. | | | The rash is seen first
on | | | the neck and upper part of | | | chest, and lasts three to | | | ten
days, when it fades and | | | the skin peels in scales, | | | flakes, or even
large | | | pieces. | |
-------------+----------------------------+-----------------------+ SMALLPOX |
Onset sudden usually with | All discharges of a | | fever and severe
backache. | patient and particles | | About third day upon | of skin or
scabs. | | subsidence of constitutional | | | symptoms red shot-like | | |
pimples, felt below the | | | skin, and seen first about | | | the face and
wrists most on | | | exposed surfaces, develop. | | | They form little
blisters | | | and after two days more | | | become filled with yellowish | |
| matter. Scabs form which | | | begin to fall off about the | | | fourteenth
day. | | -------------+----------------------------+-----------------------+ SORE
THROAT, | Begins with sore throat and | Discharges from nose |
ACUTE, | weakness. Throat diffusely | and mouth of a | SEPTIC |
reddened and may show | patient. | | patches like diphtheria. | |
-------------+----------------------------+-----------------------+ WHOOPING |
Begins with cough which is | Discharges from nose | COUGH | worse
at night. Symptoms may | and mouth of a | | at first be very mild. |
patient. | | Characteristic "whooping" | | | cough develops in about 2 | | |
weeks, and the spasm of | | | coughing sometimes ends with | | |
vomiting. | |

===
===

| EXCLUSION FROM SCHOOL |
|-------+------------------+-------------------+ | | OTHER CHILDREN |
OTHER SCHOOL | | | OF SAME | CHILDREN | DISEASE | |
HOUSEHOLD | ESPECIALLY EXPOSED | |
+---------+----------+--------+-----------+ |Patient| | | | | | | Non- | | Non- | | | |
immunes|Immunes[3]| immunes| Immunes[3]| | | | | | | |
-------------+--------+--------+----------+--------+-----------+ CHICKENPOX |
Yes | Yes | No | Yes | No |
-------------+--------+--------+----------+--------+-----------+ DIPHTHERIA | Yes
| Yes | Yes | Yes | Yes |

-------------+-------+--------+----------+--------+----------+ MEASLES | Yes |
Yes | No | Yes | No |
-------------+-------+--------+----------+--------+----------+ MEASLES | Yes |
Yes | No | Yes | No | (LIBERTY) | | | | | |
-------------+-------+--------+----------+--------+----------+ MUMPS | Yes |
Yes | No | Yes | No |
-------------+-------+--------+----------+--------+----------+ POLIOMYELITIS|
Yes | Yes | Yes | Yes | Yes |
-------------+-------+--------+----------+--------+----------+ SCARLET | Yes |
Yes | Yes | Yes | Yes | FEVER | | | | | |
-------------+-------+--------+----------+--------+----------+ SMALLPOX | Yes |
Yes | Yes | Yes | No |
-------------+-------+--------+----------+--------+----------+ SORE THROAT, |
Yes | No | No | No | No | ACUTE, | | | | | | SEPTIC | | | | | |
-------------+-------+--------+----------+--------+----------+ WHOOPING | Yes
| Yes | No | Yes | No | COUGH | | | | | |
==
==
| DURATION OF EXCLUSION FROM DATE OF ONSET |
+--------------+------------+------------------------+------------+ | | PATIENT |
PATIENT REMAINS | | | | GOES TO | ISOLATED AT | | | | HOSPITAL |
HOME | | DISEASE | +------------ ---- |-------------+------------+ | | PATIENT |
Other | Other | Children | Children | | | children | children | who leave |
exposed | | | of | who | household | at | | | the same | remain at | as
soon as | school | | | household | home | disease is | | | | | | discovered |
| ------------+--------------+------------+-----------+------------+------------+
CHICKENPOX | Until all | Exclude if non-immune until |Exclude | |
scabs are | 21st day after child last |from | | shed and | saw patient.
|school if | | disinfection | |non-immune | | of person; | |during | | at least
| |11th to 22d | | 12 days. | |days after | | | |child last | | | |saw patient.|
------------+--------------+------------------------------------+------------+
DIPHTHERIA |Until | Until two cultures at least 24 | | |patient is | hours
apart are reported | | |recovered | negative. Those showing | | |and has
two | diphtheria bacilli should not | | |cultures | necessarily be
immunized | | |from throat | unless symptoms appear. | | |and nose
which| | | |contain no | | | |diphtheria | | | |bacilli; | | | |cultures not | | | |to
be taken | | | |until 9 days | | | |from date of | | | |onset. | | | |Disinfection |
| | |of person. | | |
------------+--------------+------------------------------------+------------+

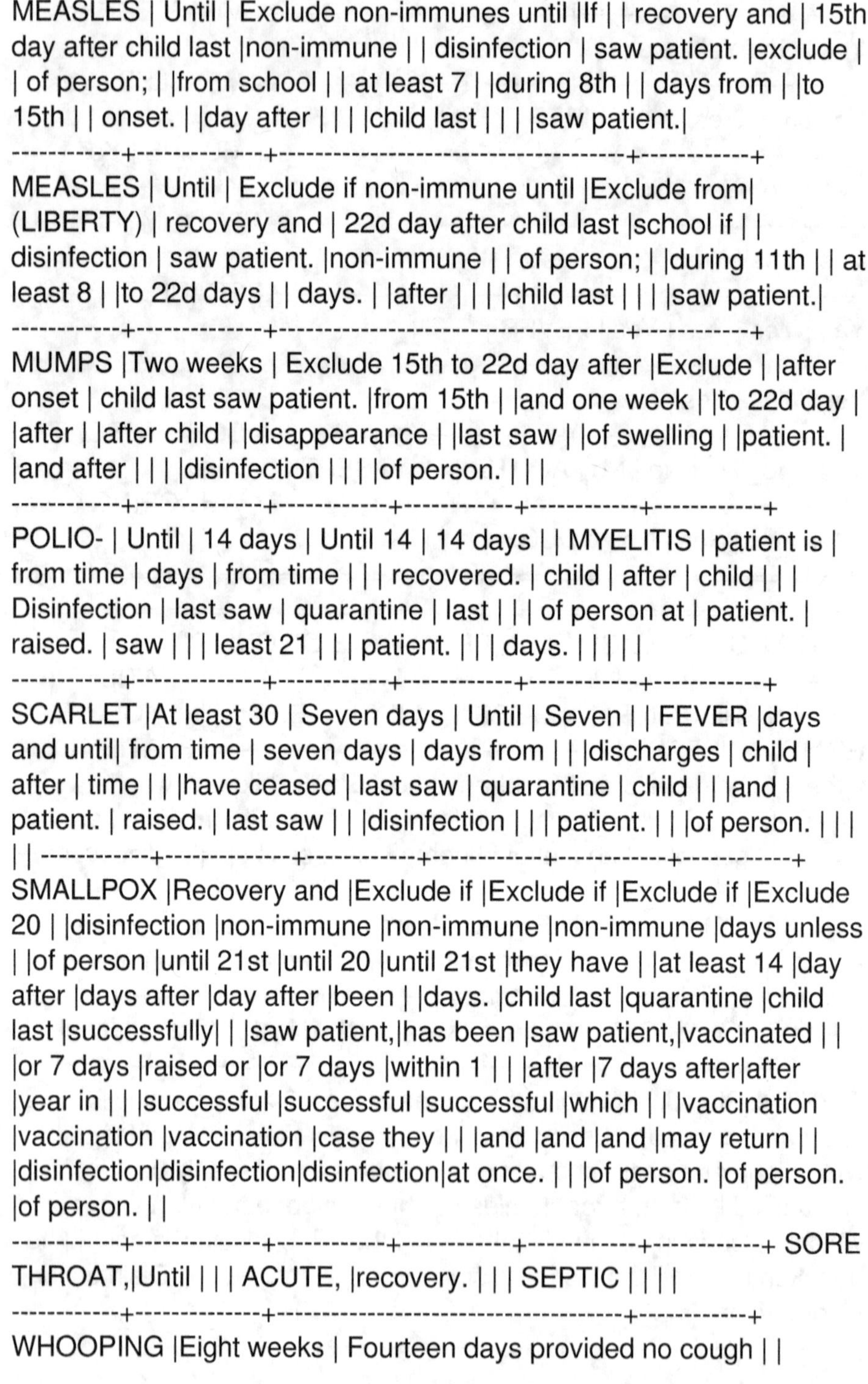

MEASLES | Until | Exclude non-immunes until |If | | recovery and | 15th day after child last |non-immune | | disinfection | saw patient. |exclude | | of person; | |from school | | at least 7 | |during 8th | | days from | |to 15th | | onset. | |day after | | | |child last | | | |saw patient.|

------------+-------------+---------------------------------------+------------+

MEASLES | Until | Exclude if non-immune until |Exclude from| (LIBERTY) | recovery and | 22d day after child last |school if | | disinfection | saw patient. |non-immune | | of person; | |during 11th | | at least 8 | |to 22d days | | days. | |after | | | |child last | | | |saw patient.|

------------+-------------+---------------------------------------+------------+

MUMPS |Two weeks | Exclude 15th to 22d day after |Exclude | |after onset | child last saw patient. |from 15th | |and one week | |to 22d day | |after | |after child | |disappearance | |last saw | |of swelling | |patient. | |and after | | | |disinfection | | | |of person. | | |

------------+-------------+------------+------------+------------+------------+

POLIO- | Until | 14 days | Until 14 | 14 days | | MYELITIS | patient is | from time | days | from time | | | recovered. | child | after | child | | | Disinfection | last saw | quarantine | last | | | of person at | patient. | raised. | saw | | | least 21 | | | patient. | | | days. | | | | |

------------+-------------+------------+------------+------------+------------+

SCARLET |At least 30 | Seven days | Until | Seven | | FEVER |days and until| from time | seven days | days from | | |discharges | child | after | time | | |have ceased | last saw | quarantine | child | | |and | patient. | raised. | last saw | | |disinfection | | | patient. | | |of person. | | | | ------------+-------------+------------+------------+------------+------------+

SMALLPOX |Recovery and |Exclude if |Exclude if |Exclude if |Exclude 20 | |disinfection |non-immune |non-immune |non-immune |days unless | |of person |until 21st |until 20 |until 21st |they have | |at least 14 |day after |days after |day after |been | |days. |child last |quarantine |child last |successfully| | |saw patient,|has been |saw patient,|vaccinated | | |or 7 days |raised or |or 7 days |within 1 | | |after |7 days after|after |year in | | |successful |successful |successful |which | | |vaccination |vaccination |vaccination |vaccination |case they | | |and |and |and |may return | | |disinfection|disinfection|disinfection|at once. | | |of person. |of person. |of person. | |

------------+-------------+------------+------------+------------+------------+ SORE THROAT,|Until | | | ACUTE, |recovery. | | | SEPTIC | | | |

------------+-------------+---------------------------------------+------------+

WHOOPING |Eight weeks | Fourteen days provided no cough | |

COUGH |or until 1 | develops. | | |week after | | | |last | | | |characteristic|
| | |cough and | | | |disinfection | | | |of person. | | |
===
===
DISEASE | Remarks | | |
-------------+---+ CHICKENPOX | A
mild disease and seldom any after effects. |
-------------+---+ DIPHTHERIA | Very
dangerous, both during attack and from | | after effects. When
diphtheria occurs in a | | school all children suffering from sore throat | |
should be excluded and the health officer | | notified. The medical
school inspector or | | health officer should take cultures from all | |
inflamed throats and noses. There is great | | variation of type, and
mild cases are often | | not recognized, but are as infectious as | |
severe cases. There is frequently no immunity | | from further attacks. |
-------------+---+ MEASLES | After
effects often severe. Period of greatest | | risk of infection three days,
before and after | | the rash appears. Great variation in type | | of
disease. Dangerous in children under 2 | | years of age. During an
outbreak all children | | having a temperature over 99°F. should | | be
sent home and the health officer notified. |
-------------+---+ MEASLES | After
effects slight. Regulations strict, | (LIBERTY) | because frequently
confused with scarlet fever. |
-------------+---+ MUMPS | Seldom
leaves after effects. Very infectious. | | Inflammation of genital organs
of male or | | female may occur. |
-------------+---+ POLIOMYELITIS|
Disease is most communicable in the early | | stages. After effect is
paralysis of certain | | muscle groups, transitory or permanent. | | Death
is due usually to paralysis of | | respiratory muscles. |
-------------+---+ SCARLET |
Dangerous both during attack and from after | FEVER | effects. Great
variation in type of disease. | | Slight attacks are as infectious as
severe | | ones. Many mild cases not diagnosed and | | many
concealed. A second attack is rare. | | When scarlet fever occurs in a
school, all | | cases of sore throat should be sent home and | | health
officer notified. Most fatal in | | children under ten years. |
-------------+---+ SMALLPOX |

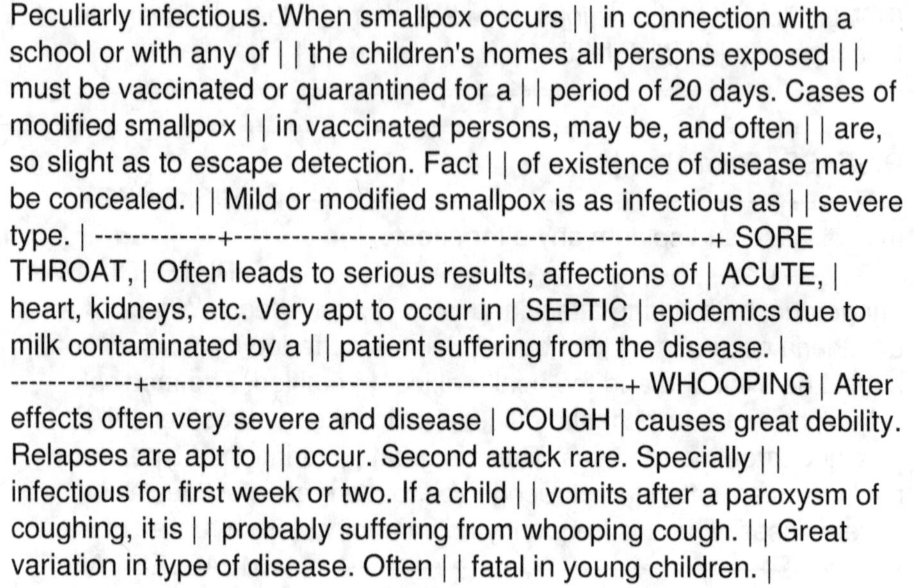

Peculiarly infectious. When smallpox occurs | | in connection with a school or with any of | | the children's homes all persons exposed | | must be vaccinated or quarantined for a | | period of 20 days. Cases of modified smallpox | | in vaccinated persons, may be, and often | | are, so slight as to escape detection. Fact | | of existence of disease may be concealed. | | Mild or modified smallpox is as infectious as | | severe type. | -------------+--+ SORE THROAT, | Often leads to serious results, affections of | ACUTE, | heart, kidneys, etc. Very apt to occur in | SEPTIC | epidemics due to milk contaminated by a | | patient suffering from the disease. | --------------+---+ WHOOPING | After effects often very severe and disease | COUGH | causes great debility. Relapses are apt to | | occur. Second attack rare. Specially | | infectious for first week or two. If a child | | vomits after a paroxysm of coughing, it is | | probably suffering from whooping cough. | | Great variation in type of disease. Often | | fatal in young children. |

===

[3] Immunes are those who have had the diseases or in smallpox, who have been successfully vaccinated within a year.

DISINFECTION: The cleansing and disinfection of the person includes washing the entire body and the hair with soap and water; thorough brushing of the teeth; rinsing the mouth; gargling the throat, and douching and spraying the nose with an antiseptic solution; and finally, a complete change of clothing (or a change of underwear and a thorough shaking and brushing of the outer garments out of doors before these are put on again). (*Facing p. 247*)

It may be added that the ways by which poliomyelitis, or infantile paralysis, is spread are not definitely known at the time of writing. We are justified, however, in believing that investigation now in progress will make exact information available in the near future.

"The weight of present opinion inclines to the view that poliomyelitis is exclusively a human disease, and is spread by personal contact, whatever other causes may be found to contribute to its spread. In personal contact we mean to include all the usual opportunities, direct or indirect, immediate or intermediate, for the transference of body discharges from person to person, having in mind as a possibility that the infection may occur through contaminated food.

"The incubation period has not been definitely established in human beings. The information at hand indicates that it is less than two weeks, and probably in the great majority of cases between 3 and 8 days."--(Report of Special Committee on Infantile Paralysis, American Journal of Public Health, November 1916.)

DISINFECTION

Specific directions for disinfecting in every kind of communicable disease would be too extended to be given here. In each case the attendant should learn from the doctor just how that particular disease is communicated, just what discharges, utensils, linen, etc., need to be disinfected, and just what disinfectants he prefers to have used. The following general methods are now in use, but it must be remembered that from time to time new methods are devised and new disinfectants are discovered.

CARE OF NOSE AND THROAT DISCHARGES.--The care of handkerchiefs has already been described on page 239. Cloths or cotton used to wipe the eyes or to receive any other bodily discharge including vomitus, should be collected in the same way and burned. Everyone should be taught in early childhood to cover the nose and mouth with a handkerchief during coughing and sneezing; if the patient has not already learned to do so he must be taught now. If the amount of expectoration is great, waterproof receptacles should be provided, which should be burned with their contents.

CARE OF DISCHARGES FROM THE BOWELS AND BLADDER.--At the present time the following preparations are commonly used to disinfect stools and urine: 5% solution of carbolic acid; chloride of lime solution, made freshly whenever needed by mixing thoroughly ½ pound of chloride of lime with one gallon of water; and unslaked lime to which is added *hot* water. The amount of carbolic solution used should be about equal in bulk to the amount of material to be disinfected; the chloride of lime solution should be at least twice, and the unslaked lime at least one-eighth the bulk. Fecal masses should be broken up so that the disinfectant may reach every part; they may be stirred with tightly twisted toilet paper, which should be left in the bedpan and disinfected with the stools. If these substances are used, disinfection is considered complete at the end of an hour, and the contents of the bedpan may then be emptied into the toilet with safety. It may be necessary to provide two bedpans so that one may be available for use while the contents of the other is being disinfected. Bedpans and urinals should be boiled daily and kept thoroughly clean at all times.

In places having no sewerage system, disinfected discharges may be emptied into a trench situated at a distance from the well, and then covered with earth. As an extra precaution, the disinfected discharges may be mixed with sawdust or kerosene and burned in the trench. Directions for installing a sanitary privy may be found in Bulletin 68 of the United States Public Health Service.

BATH WATER and water that has been used for cleansing the teeth and mouth may be disinfected in the same way as urine, or it may be emptied into a suitable receptacle and boiled ten minutes.

CARE OF THE HANDS.--Disinfectants for the hands should be used in addition to scrubbing with soap and water, not as a substitute. The hands may be disinfected after scrubbing by soaking them for three minutes in one of the following solutions: alcohol 70%, carbolic acid solution 2½%, or a solution made by adding one teaspoonful of lysol or of creolin to a pint of water. These disinfectants are poisons if taken internally; the bottles must be carefully labeled and kept in a safe place. It is a good plan to wear rubber gloves when handling infective material; the gloves should afterward be boiled for ten minutes.

CARE OF UTENSILS.--A sufficient number of dishes, spoons, tumblers, basins, etc. must be reserved for the patient's exclusive use; these utensils must be washed separately and dried with towels not used for other dishes. Mistakes frequently occur by which other persons use the patient's dishes, and in consequence his dishes should not be kept in the cupboard with other dishes; if no other safe place can be found, they had better stay in the patient's room covered with a clean cloth or napkin. The dishes should be scalded daily and at the termination of the illness they must be boiled briskly for ten minutes before they are returned to general use. Food left on the patient's tray should be burned; it should not be eaten by any one else, nor placed in the pantry or refrigerator with other food.

CARE OF LINEN.--A satisfactory way to disinfect towels, night gowns, bed linen, etc. is to place the articles immediately in a wash boiler filled with cold water to which a little washing soda has been added, and then to boil them in the same water for twenty minutes; they can afterward go safely into the regular laundry. The boiling may be done once a day; articles soiled in the meantime may be left to soak in the cold water and soda.

DISINFECTION OF THE PERSON.--"The cleansing and disinfection of the person includes washing the entire body and the hair with soap and water; thorough brushing of the teeth; rinsing the mouth; gargling the throat, and douching and spraying the nose with an antiseptic solution; and finally, a complete change of clothing (or a change of underwear) and a thorough shaking and brushing of the outer garments out-of-doors before these are put on again."--(New York State Department of Health.)

TERMINATION OF QUARANTINE.--After the patient has recovered, he and the attendant should, if the doctor thinks it necessary, disinfect themselves as directed above before they mingle again with other people. The exact time when it is safe for a person to come out of quarantine and resume ordinary life varies in different diseases. Moreover, opinion differs in regard to quarantine periods for the same diseases, so that the regulations of Boards of Health in different cities show wide variations. It is of course impossible to say at just what moment every patient, or even the majority of patients, will stop expelling germs. Quarantine periods are intended to protect the community as completely as possible without causing unnecessary hardship to individuals. In any given case, the local regulations should be strictly observed but release from quarantine is not a guarantee that the patient is not still discharging germs, and extreme care should still be taken to prevent the spread of saliva and other discharges.

TERMINAL DISINFECTION.--A room that has been occupied by a patient with a communicable disease should be thoroughly cleaned at the termination of the illness. Dishes, utensils, bed linen, etc. should be cared for in the ways already described. The floor, bedstead, and other furniture should be washed with hot water, soap, and washing soda. The walls, windows, etc., should be wiped with a cloth wrung out of hot water, soap suds, and soda. The mattress, unless badly soiled with discharges, should be scrubbed with the same solution and a stiff brush, and left out-of-doors in the sunshine for a day or two, or until dry. If badly soiled, it is best to destroy the mattress unless the Board of Health has facilities for steam sterilization. Ordinary washing is all that is generally required for blankets, but if badly soiled they should be sterilized by steam or burned. The room should then be thoroughly sunned and aired for a day or two, with the windows wide open both day and night. Sunning and airing are among the most important measures in disinfecting a room, and should not be slighted. If there has been gross pollution, as when a careless consumptive persists in spitting on the floor and walls, it may be necessary to remove the old paint and paper and have the room done over. The room may safely be occupied after all these measures have been taken.

FUMIGATION.--Many Boards of Health have abandoned fumigation after communicable diseases, except after those which like typhus and yellow fever, are carried by vermin or insects. Dry formaldehyde gas, which was formerly used for fumigation, has a violent effect on mucous membranes, but its power to kill bacteria, even on surfaces, appears to be weak, while its penetrating power is not sufficient to disinfect bedding, carpets, upholstered furniture, and other fabrics. Since fumigation is costly, troublesome, and ineffectual there seems to be no good reason for using it. Moreover, its use gives a false sense of security, so that really effective measures like sunning, airing, and scrubbing are likely to be neglected.

Theory and practice of disinfection, it is clear, have radically changed in recent years. Modern knowledge requires concurrent disinfection, or the destruction of germs from the moment when symptoms are first noticed; all the time, day and night, this disinfection must go on with unremitting care. Today wet sheets are not hung in doorways nor are chemicals left about in open dishes to disinfect quite harmless air, but scrupulous cleanliness at all stages of disease is recognized as one of the most important measures, if not the most important measure, in disinfection.

EXERCISES

1. Summarize the ways in which infectious diseases are spread.

2. What is meant by the incubation period? State the length of the incubation period in measles; Liberty measles; whooping-cough; scarlet fever; chicken-pox; diphtheria; mumps; typhoid fever.

3. Name some of the early symptoms common to most infectious diseases. If such symptoms appear, what should be done while waiting for the doctor to come?

4. Discuss the importance, prevention, and treatment of common colds.

5. What measures should be taken to isolate a patient who is suffering from a communicable disease?

6. What special care should the attendant of a patient with a communicable disease give to her own clothing and person?

7. Why are the children's diseases more serious in reality than they are commonly supposed to be?

8. Describe the symptoms of each of the following: Measles, scarlet fever, chicken-pox, mumps, whooping-cough, and diphtheria.

9. How should bowel and bladder discharges be disinfected?

10. How should dishes and other utensils be disinfected?

11. How should linen be disinfected?

12. Describe measures necessary for concurrent disinfection.

13. Describe measures necessary for terminal disinfection.

FOR FURTHER READING

Preventive Medicine and Hygiene--Rosenau.

The New Public Health--Hill, Chapters VII-XVII.

Essentials of Medicine--Emerson, Chapters XII-XV.

Health and Disease--Roger I. Lee, Chapter X-XIV.

Disease and Its Causes--Councilman, Chapters V-IX.

Publications of the New York State Department of Health, Albany, entitled: The Teacher and Communicable Disease; A Method for the Control of Communicable Diseases in Schools; Regulations and Instructions for Cleansing and Disinfection; The Conduct of an Isolation Period for Communicable Disease in a Home; Tuberculosis; Typhoid Fever; Scarlet Fever; Measles; Whooping-cough; Diphtheria; Poliomyelitis, Acute Anterior (Infantile Paralysis); Smallpox; Septic Sore Throat; Venereal Diseases. (Any of the above pamphlets will be sent upon receipt of a three cent stamp.)

CHAPTER XIII

COMMON AILMENTS AND EMERGENCIES

This chapter describes a few home treatments for the relief of slight ailments and injuries, together with some measures that may be employed in emergencies. For more extended instructions in these subjects the student should consult the Red Cross Text-book on First Aid.

CONDITIONS IN WHICH THE NERVOUS SYSTEM IS INVOLVED

HEADACHE.--Headache is not a disease in itself, but a symptom common to many different disorders. Among the abnormal conditions often causing headaches are fatigue, eyestrain, indigestion, constipation, neuralgia, rheumatism, anæmia, acute infections, and other disorders. Treatment should consist in finding the cause and removing it if possible; clearly no one remedy can cure so many different causes. A physician should be consulted if headaches are of frequent occurrence, but in many cases rest and attention to other hygienic requirements are all that is needed. During an attack of headache a hot foot bath may give relief, or a mustard paste or cold applications on the back of the neck, or an ice bag or cold compress on the forehead.

SLEEPLESSNESS, like headache, has many possible causes, and effective treatment consists in finding and removing them. Pain or discomfort of any kind, fatigue, overwork, and worry are common causes. Sleeplessness easily becomes a habit that may persist after its cause has been removed; hence a person who has formed the habit of sleeplessness should patiently strive to break the old habit and to substitute a better. A careful hygienic régime is essential for the patient, exercise in the open air, and cultivation of a hopeful and tranquil spirit. The diet should be liberal, but light and unstimulating; tea and coffee should be omitted, certainly during the latter part of the day. The patient should spend rather a dull evening, avoiding excitement and mental exertion that is difficult, even though pleasurable. He should retire early. A hot tub or foot bath, and a hot drink at bed time may help to produce sleep. The bedroom should be dark, cool, and well ventilated, the bed comfortable and the covers light but warm. The patient should be told that rest is the most important thing for him, and that he should not try too hard to sleep nor worry if unsuccessful. The patient should try to banish from his mind, at bed time, thoughts that are distressing, and even those that are especially interesting. By using patience and persistence most persons can regain the power of sleeping even when habits of sleeplessness have been long established.

FAINTING is a partial or total loss of consciousness due to a diminished supply of blood in the brain. It may follow bleeding, exhaustion from heat, fatigue from prolonged standing and the like, or strong emotional disturbance, like fear or surprise. Fainting is less common than it formerly was; it now occurs most frequently among persons suffering from anæmia, heart weakness, or special susceptibility.

Symptoms of fainting are pale face, cold perspiration, rapid, feeble pulse, and shallow, sighing respiration. Treatment consists in removing the patient into cool, fresh air, applying cold water to the face and keeping the head low. For a person who feels faint but has not lost consciousness, this treatment will probably prove sufficient; if, however, he becomes unconscious, place him so that the head is lower than the body, loosen the clothing, especially the clothing about the neck, apply cold water to the face and chest, and see that fresh air is plentiful. When the patient is sufficiently conscious to swallow, give a teaspoonful of aromatic spirits of ammonia in half a glass of water and keep him quiet until he has entirely recovered.

A person who is unconscious from any cause always requires immediate attention. In emergency work elevate the patient's head if his face is flushed, and keep it low if his face is pale. Do not try to arouse an unconscious patient by shaking him and calling to him, in the first place because it is useless to do so, and in the second, because consciousness will return spontaneously if his condition improves.

CONVULSIONS.--In every case of convulsions a doctor is needed at the earliest possible moment. Convulsions in adults are very serious;

in babies and small children although serious they are less alarming, since they may follow comparatively slight disturbances, particularly disturbances of digestion.

Treatment for babies and children with convulsions consists first in keeping the child as quiet as possible, and next in measures to draw blood from the brain toward the surface of the body. The child should first be undressed, moving him as little as possible, and put to bed between warm blankets. Cold should be applied to his head by a compress or ice bag, and hot water bag should be placed near his feet. An enema should then be given. A warm tub bath is sometimes used to apply heat, if the convulsion has not subsided by the time the child is undressed. If the bath is given the temperature of the water should not be above 106°, and should be tested by a thermometer. If no thermometer is available, the water should be tested with the elbow rather than the hand, and cold water should be added if it feels uncomfortably warm. There is great danger of scalding a child during the excitement inevitably caused by a convulsion.

Although haste is needed when a child has convulsions, yet quiet is essential, since the slightest movement tends to increase the convulsions or to start them again. As soon as the convulsions are over the child should be removed from the bath and put to bed between warm blankets. Even after the symptoms have completely subsided, the greatest care should be taken to keep the child quiet. He should be handled and disturbed as little as possible. The bath should be repeated if convulsions begin again. The doctor, when he comes, will probably order a dose of castor oil; and therefore, if It is impossible to obtain a doctor at once, the dose should be given.

SHOCK (in the medical sense of the word) or *collapse*, is a serious condition in which a patient's vitality and all his bodily processes are profoundly depressed. Generally shock occurs only after a severe injury or a long exhausting illness. Since, however, some persons are peculiarly susceptible to it, the possibility of shock must be kept in mind in treating even slight injuries. The probability of shock is somewhat increased if patients are allowed to see their own wounds. Injured persons should always sit or lie down while wounds, however slight, are dressed.

Symptoms of shock are pallor, pinched, anxious expression, dilated pupils, cold clammy skin, feeble breathing, and rapid, weak pulse. The patient may be mentally normal, or irrational, or unconscious, but more frequently he appears stupid, and though conscious, he pays no attention to what is going on. Unfortunately this condition is sometimes mistaken for sleepiness, and he is left alone to sleep just when active measures are most needed.

If a patient shows any symptom of shock the doctor should be summoned immediately, but no time should be lost in beginning treatment, since the condition may be critical. It should be remembered, however, that panic and confusion may alarm a patient who is conscious, and thus increase the shock. The patient should be covered warmly, and undressed under blankets, without exposure or avoidable moving. His head should be low, and as quickly as possible hot water bags should be placed near but not upon him. If the patient is conscious and able to swallow he should be given hot coffee or aromatic spirits of ammonia, one teaspoonful in half a glass of water. The legs and arms should be rubbed from the extremities toward the heart, but care should be taken to avoid touching or moving injured parts. The patient should stay in bed, warmly covered and closely watched for some time after he has apparently recovered.

Helping a patient into bed is not necessarily the first thing to be done in every case of sudden illness. Great harm may be done by the injudicious moving of injured persons, and often it is safer to make a person comfortable with pillows and blankets where he happens to be, certainly until a sufficient number of people can be found to lift him properly. Clothing should be removed carefully, and one should not hesitate to cut it away if undressing is painful or necessitates much moving.

STIMULANTS, in emergency work, are frequently misused. They should not be given when the head has been injured, when bleeding is profuse, or when the face is red and the pulse strong. Neither should attempts be made to give fluids of any kind to patients not sufficiently conscious to swallow. Safe stimulants to use are black coffee, tea, or aromatic spirits of ammonia. Alcoholic liquors should not be given unless prescribed by a physician.

SUNSTROKE AND HEAT EXHAUSTION are both caused by excessive heat either indoors or out, but they differ both in symptoms and in treatment.

Sunstroke or heat stroke, usually begins with acute pain in the head, followed almost immediately by loss of consciousness. The skin is dry and very hot, the face is red or purple, the pupils are dilated, the breathing is difficult, the pulse is slow, and the temperature high.

Treatment consists in sending for the doctor, removing the patient to a cool place, undressing him and applying cold, especially to the head and spine, or still better, placing him in a very cold bath. The body should be rubbed constantly in the direction of the heart. Stimulants should not be given.

Symptoms of heat exhaustion, on the other hand, resemble those of shock. The doctor should be summoned, and the patient should be removed to a cool and quiet place, where he should stay warmly covered in a reclining position. Stimulants should be given, hot water bags applied, and the other measures for treating shock should be employed.

CONDITIONS IN WHICH THE DIGESTIVE TRACT IS AFFECTED

NAUSEA AND VOMITING are frequently caused by injudicious eating, especially when a person is worried or fatigued. A doctor should be consulted if either one occurs often, or if vomiting is accompanied by pain, prostration, diarrhoea, fever, or other acute symptoms. A person who is nauseated should lie down in a cool, quiet place. Hot fomentations may be applied to the abdomen, or a mustard paste over the stomach. Soda mints or a teaspoonful of baking soda may be given dissolved in hot water, and unless diarrhoea is present a Seidlitz powder or other saline cathartic may be given. A large quantity of warm water may be given to wash out the stomach; it is more effectual if salt or mustard is added, in the proportion of one teaspoonful to a glass of water.

HICCOUGH, which is usually caused by digestive disturbances, is not serious in healthy people, and can generally be stopped by holding the breath, or by drinking water. If these measures are not effectual, salt or mustard in water as already described or a teaspoonful of the syrup of ipecac, may be given to produce vomiting. If the hiccough still continues, medical advice should be obtained.

DIARRHOEA is ordinarily caused by an infection, or by an offending substance in the intestines. The offending substance should be removed before attempts are made to check the diarrhoea. When a baby has diarrhoea four things should be done--all food should be withheld; boiled water should be given freely; bowel movements should be saved for the doctor to see; and unless a doctor can be found immediately, castor oil should be given, from one-half to one teaspoonful according to the age of the child. Similar treatment should be given to older children. Adults should take one tablespoonful of castor oil and drink boiled water freely, but they should take no food until the doctor comes.

CONSTIPATION has been discussed on pages 193 and 52.

COLIC is a sharp, intermittent pain in the abdominal region; it is caused in many instances by indigestion or chilling. The following remedies may relieve it: a hot water bag, an emetic, as salt or mustard in luke-warm water, a Seidlitz powder or other saline cathartic, soda mints, or a teaspoonful of syrup of ginger in hot water. Unless it feels sore or tender, the abdomen may be rubbed up, on the right side, across, just below the waist, and down, on the left side. Babies may be given a few teaspoonfuls of warm water, or an enema of salt and water.

Colic may be serious. The doctor should be summoned at once if the patient seems exhausted, if the pain is severe, if pain is increased rather than relieved by pressure, if the abdomen feels sore, especially on the right side, or if sharp abdominal pain is accompanied by fever, vomiting, and stubborn constipation. If the above-mentioned symptoms are present, no food, drink, or medicine should be given until the doctor comes.

CONDITIONS IN WHICH THE EYES OR EARS ARE AFFECTED

STYES generally accompany eyestrain or poor general health. The cause should be found and treated; and especial attention should be given to correcting eyestrain, indigestion, and constipation. Hot applications may be used, but if pus gathers, the stye should be treated by a physician.

FOREIGN BODIES IN THE EYE may sometimes be removed by blowing the nose violently, by yawning several times, or by drawing the upper lid down over the lower. The eye should not be rubbed. If it proves impossible to dislodge the object by these methods or by others similar, the patient's eyelid should be turned back in the following way: Let the patient sit with his head back in a low chair placed in a good light, and stand behind him holding his head between your side and upper arm. In this position the patient's head is held firmly while both of the operator's hands are free. Next draw down the lower lid, and remove the object, if visible, on the corner of a clean handkerchief. To turn back the upper lid, grasp the eyelashes firmly, draw the lid down, out, and then up over a match or pencil placed across the middle line of the lid and held in your other hand. Then wipe the object carefully away if it is visible.

Irritation that persists after the foreign body has been removed may be relieved by a cold compress continued for an hour or more, or by a drop or two of castor oil placed under the lid. If attempts to remove the foreign body prove unsuccessful, if the injury is severe, or if irritation continues after several hours, apply a cold compress, bandage it firmly so that the eyeball is kept at rest, and seek the aid of a physician.

DISORDERS AFFECTING THE EARS.--Permanent deafness may result from neglecting disorders of the ears. Ear-ache, discharge from the ear, swelling in or about it, pain or tenderness behind it, all require medical attention and no time should be lost in securing it. To relieve pain the patient may lie with the ear on an ice bag, but nothing whatever should be put into the ear before the doctor comes, except when an insect has entered the ear, and causes acute distress by the noise of its beating wings. If such an accident has occurred, the patient should lie on the unaffected side, and warm sweet oil should be dropped very gently into the affected ear by means of a medicine dropper. The insect generally drowns in the oil and floats to the opening of the ear canal. After it has been removed, the patient should lie on the affected side so that the oil may drain out of the ear.

No attempts should be made to remove foreign bodies from the ear or nose, unless they can be reached easily with the fingers. Hair pins, crochet hooks and similar instruments should never be used for this purpose. It is best for a doctor to remove foreign objects because unskillful attempts are likely to move them further in.

CONDITIONS IN WHICH THE SKIN IS AFFECTED

PRICKLY-HEAT, which affects babies and children more often than adults, is an eruption caused by heat and moisture, and aggravated by flannel underwear. It may be prevented by keeping the skin dry and cool, and it may be relieved by bathing the skin with alcohol and water, about one part of alcohol to three of water, and by using after the bath a powder made of two parts of starch to one of boracic acid, or any good talcum powder.

INSECT BITES AND STINGS.--The sting, if still in the wound, should first be removed, and then ammonia should be applied, since the poison is generally acid. Applications of cold water, alcohol and water, or wet salt may relieve the subsequent burning and itching, but ammonia is generally most effective.

IVY POISONING may be treated by applying cloths wet in a strong solution of baking soda or of boracic acid, or by applications of carbolized vaseline or ichthyol. Severe cases should have medical attention. Scratching and rubbing seem to spread the inflammation, and special care should be taken not to rub the face or eyes with infected hands. Susceptible people should avoid the plant if possible.

OTHER EMERGENCIES

CHILLS may be the result of infection or of exposure to cold. An early diagnosis of the trouble is so desirable that it is well to send for a doctor even when symptoms are not severe. If a person has a chill his temperature should be taken at once; fever and chill together probably indicate invasion by bacteria. When chills follow exposure to cold the patient should go to bed between warm blankets, his body should be briskly rubbed, and hot water bags and a hot drink should be given. If he prefers, he may take a hot bath before going to bed.

CROUP is caused by a spasmodic closure of the larynx so that breathing is impeded. The child who develops croup may have a slight cold, but frequently shows no symptoms until he wakes in the night with a hoarse ringing cough and difficult breathing. True croup, though often distressing, is seldom serious, even when the symptoms are so severe that the child appears to be partly suffocated. An emetic should be given at once, preferably syrup of ipecac, one teaspoonful followed by warm water, or ten drops every 15 minutes until the child vomits freely. Hot fomentations may be applied to the throat and chest in order to hasten relaxation of the muscular spasm, and water should be kept boiling near the bed in a teakettle or uncovered saucepan. The child should stay in a warm room during the following day.

Whenever a child develops a croupy cough his throat should be examined. A physician should be summoned if the throat is red and especially if the redness is associated with rise in temperature. Cases of diphtheria have been overlooked by neglecting such symptoms.

BLEEDING

In the vast majority of cases, bleeding can be stopped by elevating the injured part and applying pressure over the wound. One should, however, remember that loss of blood is not the only danger presented by an open wound, for pus-producing germs, if they make their entrance, may cause an infection which may be as serious as the bleeding itself. Hence in dealing with open wounds of any sort one should always keep in mind the danger of infection as well as the danger from loss of blood.

TREATMENT OF SLIGHT WOUNDS.--Loss of blood from slight wounds is seldom so serious as the danger of infection; therefore small cuts, pin pricks, scratches, etc. should be encouraged to bleed by pressure near the wound in order to expel the germs that may have entered. After the wound has bled a little, tincture of iodine should be applied by means of a cotton swab both to the wound itself and also to the surrounding skin.

After the wound has thus been disinfected it should be covered with a sterile dressing; a sterile or aseptic dressing is material in which all bacterial life has been destroyed. Gauze from a First Aid dressing or from a packet of sterile gauze should be used for this compress, or gauze may be cut from a sterile bandage. The compress serves two purposes: it protects the wound from infection, and if applied with pressure it checks further bleeding.

The compress should be securely bandaged in place, or its edges may be fastened with adhesive plaster or collodion. Neither of the two latter should cover the wound itself. The outside bandage may be changed when soiled, but the compress itself should not be disturbed until the wound has healed. It is a mistake to dress wounds oftener than necessary, since handling them always increases the chance of introducing germs. Most children, like Tom Sawyer, delight in wounds, but they should be prevented if possible both from inspecting and from exhibiting them.

If heat, swelling, redness, or pain develop in a wound after a day or two, a doctor should be consulted; and not a minute should be lost if the patient has a chill or if red streaks appear extending from the wound in the general direction of the heart. Until the doctor comes the wounded part should be elevated and covered with cold applications wet in alcohol 25%, or in a solution of common salt, a teaspoonful to a pint of water.

Several points should be remembered in dressing wounds. In the first place the mouth, which is full of germs, is not a good place for cut fingers. Moreover, wounds should not be touched by anything, especially the fingers, either washed or unwashed, nor should the scissors, fingers or other object be allowed to touch the surface of the dressing that is to be placed directly upon a wound. Unless they contain gross dirt wounds should not be washed with water, since washing introduces another chance of infection and accomplishes nothing except a tidy appearance, which is not essential. Furthermore, it should be remembered that exposure to the air will not infect a wound, and therefore time should be taken to find a suitable dressing.

When a sterile dressing is quite impossible to obtain, the cleanest material available should be used; one of the best substitutes for a sterile dressing is the inner surface of a handkerchief or napkin that has not previously been unfolded since it was ironed. It is a common mistake to tie up a wound in the first article presented, which is usually a generous by-stander's soiled handkerchief. The same precautions in regard to cleanliness should be taken in dressing wounds that are known to be contaminated, since even into an infected wound it is possible to introduce more germs and more virulent ones.

NOSEBLEED usually stops of itself, but if it is obstinate the patient should sit erect with the head back, and cold compresses should be placed on the nose and at the back of the neck. Pressure should be made on the upper lip by means of the fingers, or by a firm roll of paper or cotton placed under the upper lip. Salt or vinegar in water, a teaspoonful of either one to a cup of water, may be snuffed up the nose. The treatment should be continued for ten or fifteen minutes, or until bleeding stops; if the bleeding persists a doctor is needed.

PROFUSE MENSTRUATION should be treated by keeping the patient quiet in bed with the head low and the feet slightly elevated. "Any marked increase, whether by amount, duration, or shortening of the interval between the periods ought to receive attention and be brought to the physician's notice" (Latimer). Painful menstruation may be relieved by rest in bed, mental as well as physical, by hot drinks and by the application of heat. Rest, and hygienic living persistently practised, will relieve most menstrual abnormalities. The common practice of using patent remedies and alcoholic liquors for disordered menstruation cannot be too strongly condemned.

OTHER INJURIES

SPRAINS.--A sprain is caused by twisting, stretching, or tearing the tissues about a joint. The first sharp pain comes from the injury to the tissues; subsequent pain is caused by the pressure of accumulated fluid. The other symptoms are those characteristic of inflammation.

When a sprain is slight, the affected part should be elevated and kept at rest for the first twenty-four hours. Either heat or cold should be applied, or heat and cold alternately; a good treatment is to soak the part in hot water and afterward to allow cold water to run upon it from the tap. Gentle rubbing with a circular motion helps to reduce the swelling. If the joint must be used it should be bandaged tightly.

Injuries to joints should never be neglected; and severe sprains always require medical attention, since in addition to the sprain a bone may be broken. A severely sprained joint should be elevated, treated with hot or cold applications, and kept at rest until it has been examined by a physician.

BRUISES.--Bruises need no attention unless they are extensive or painful. The skin should be kept clean and if possible unbroken, since injured tissues are less resistant to infection than tissues in their normal state. Applications of cold water or of equal parts of cold water and alcohol may relieve the pain, but cold should not be used upon bruises that are extensive. A compress bandaged tightly in place may help to prevent swelling and discoloration.

BURNS AND SCALDS.--Injuries from dry heat are called burns, and those from moist heat are called scalds. Both are painful, and both are dangerous if extensive or deep. Burns and scalds require medical attention if the injured area is extensive, if a large blister is formed, if the skin is destroyed or charred, and if symptoms of shock appear. Shock often follows burns or scalds even when the injury is comparatively slight.

Treatment of slight burns, where the skin is reddened but not destroyed, has for its main object the exclusion of air. One of the following may be applied: dry baking soda, or baking soda made into a paste with water, picric acid gauze moistened in water, boracic acid ointment, vaseline, sweet oil, or castor oil; if none of these is obtainable, lard, cream, the white of an egg or unsalted butter may be used. Old muslin or linen bandaged lightly in place, should be used to cover the burn.

The same treatment is used for sunburn, and also for small burns where blisters form. A blister, if it forms, should not be punctured; but if it is accidentally broken the skin of the blister should not be removed. It should be remembered that a broken blister is an open wound, and therefore liable to infection.

BRUSH BURN is a name given to injuries where the surface of the skin has been removed. They include the scraped arms and legs which are common accidents in childhood. In order to dress a brush burn, particles of dirt should first be removed preferably by means of forceps that have been boiled, and the surrounding skin should then be cleansed with soap and water. The injured part should next be flushed with sterile salt solution, made by boiling water five minutes and adding to it salt in the proportion of one teaspoonful to a pint of water. If the dirt is difficult to remove a soap compress should be applied. To prepare the compress several thicknesses of gauze or muslin should be boiled in a strong solution of castile or green soap for ten minutes. The compress should remain in place several hours, and may be repeated if necessary. After the wound has been thoroughly cleansed, it should be dressed with old muslin that has been saturated in castor oil or spread with boracic ointment.

EXERCISES

1. Name some common causes of headache and of sleeplessness, and outline rational treatment for each of these disorders.

2. Describe symptoms and treatment of shock; of fainting; of convulsions in children.

3. Describe the treatment of all disturbances of the digestive tract mentioned in this book.

4. What should be done if a foreign body has entered the eye? if one has entered the ear? What should be done for a person who has a stye? for a person with pain in or near the ear?

5. How would you treat a sprain?

6. Describe treatment for burns and scalds.

7. Distinguish between heat stroke and heat prostration, and tell what treatment should be given in each case.

8. What are the two principal dangers from slight wounds, and how should one guard against them? Show how you would dress a small cut.

9. What should you do for a person with nose bleed?

FOR FURTHER READING

American National Red Cross Text Book on First Aid--Lynch.

Immediate Care of the Injured--Morrow.

Prompt Aid to the Injured--Doty.

CHAPTER XIV

SPECIAL POINTS IN THE CARE OF CHILDREN, CONVALESCENTS, CHRONICS, AND THE AGED

In many cases of sickness institutional care has marked advantages. It may be the only solution when adequate provision for the sick is impossible at home; and it is often a necessity when a patient requires special equipment or apparatus, expert nursing, and medical attention within reach both day and night.

On the other hand, it would not be desirable even if it were possible for all sick persons to be cared for in institutions. Care at home when it is adequate may be more successful than equally skillful care given elsewhere, since the sick quite as much as the well are injured by long separation from normal family life. Most children, because they need the attention of their own mothers, most convalescent and chronic patients, and most aged persons are cared for at home; and in the great majority of cases no better place for them could be found. Since patients of these four groups have needs peculiar to themselves, some special points in caring for them are considered in this chapter.

CHILDREN

Ability to observe quickly and accurately is seldom more needed than it is by a woman who cares for children. No one expects babies to explain their troubles, but people forget that small children are unable to describe their physical sensations with any degree of accuracy, although discomfort or sickness may show itself in all degrees of ill temper and bad conduct. For these exhibitions many a suffering child has been punished, where an older and more articulate person would have received considerate attention.

Children, like babies, have a low resistance to disease. Moreover, they react quickly both to favorable and to unfavorable surroundings. Hence slight causes sometimes produce pronounced or even violent symptoms in children without giving cause for great anxiety, although the same symptoms if exhibited by adults, might indicate critical illness. On the other hand the recuperative power of children is high, and their recoveries are sometimes surprisingly rapid. It is a mistake, when a child has completely recovered from an acute but brief illness, to coddle him for weeks afterward merely because a grown person in similar circumstances would have failed to regain his strength.

When a child is sick in bed, especial efforts should be made to insure adequate ventilation without chilling him. Children always lose heat rapidly because the body surface is proportionately large; when they are ill, therefore, it is especially necessary to keep them well covered, to see that their hands and feet are warm, and to avoid chilling them during their baths. But overheating must also be avoided, since all children, sick or well, who are too warmly dressed or who stay in rooms that are too warm, become weak and irritable and more susceptible than others to colds and other respiratory disorders. The child's skin should be kept clean and dry, but he should not be disturbed nor handled unnecessarily.

Sick children require very simple food at short intervals. Variety is not so necessary for a child as for an adult, unless the child has been allowed to form bad habits of eating. Sick children should not be indulged unnecessarily, either in regard to their food or in other ways. However, attempts made during an illness to change the habits of a badly trained child are unwise because usually unsuccessful; parents who sow the wind by neglecting to train their children when they are in good health may as well make up their minds to reap a veritable whirlwind when the children are ill. Even when children are well trained it is difficult and sometimes impossible to prevent them from forming bad habits during sickness. Yet the labor of training a child reaps perhaps at no other time a richer reward than it does when the child is ill, and his recovery might be seriously impeded by unwillingness to accept necessary food, medicine, or treatment.

PHYSICAL DEFECTS are faults in the structure of the body; adenoid growths, imperfect eyes, abnormally curved spines, and defective teeth are examples. Most physical defects can be cured in childhood by treatment or by slight operations. If untreated they frequently lead to sickness or to serious impairment of the body, and if neglected until adult life their injurious consequences are generally beyond remedy, even when the defects themselves can be repaired.

Some indications of common physical defects are given below; they ought to be more generally known than they are. If a child exhibits one or more of the symptoms mentioned, he ought to be given a complete physical examination by a competent physician, and treatment, if needed, should begin without delay. The idea that children will outgrow these defects without treatment is erroneous. Better, however, than waiting until symptoms appear is the modern way of giving every child a physical examination at stated intervals, a practice already common in public schools where effective health work is carried on.

EYESTRAIN frequently comes from imperfections in the shape of the eye; these imperfections can almost always be corrected by glasses. When a child is suffering from eyestrain, the eyes themselves may show indications of trouble; they may be blood-shot, the lids may itch or be crusted or inflamed, or styes may appear. In other cases the symptoms of eyestrain have no apparent connection with the eyes; such symptoms are headache, nausea, vomiting, indigestion, fatigue, irritability, poor scholarship, and nervous exhaustion. If a child shows any of these symptoms, or if he rubs his eyes, frowns, squints, wrinkles his forehead, sits bent over his book, or develops round shoulders, there is sufficient reason for having his eyes examined by an oculist. Examination by an optician should not be considered sufficient.

ENLARGED TONSILS AND ADENOIDS.--The tonsils are masses of spongy tissue situated at the back of the mouth, on either side of the opening into the throat. If enlarged they may seriously interfere with breathing, and if diseased they frequently harbor the germs causing many acute infections, as well as germs of rheumatism and most of the heart disease originating in early life. Therefore the tonsils ought to be removed if they are diseased or greatly enlarged, but there is ordinarily no good reason for removing normal tonsils.

Adenoids are situated at the back of the nose, and like the tonsils are composed of spongy tissue. Adenoids sometimes become so enlarged that they interfere with the passage of air through the nose, thus predisposing to catarrh, colds, and other respiratory diseases, to high palate with irregular teeth, to inflammation of the middle ear leading to deafness, to diminished mental activity, and to general poor health.

If a child breathes through his mouth, if he snores at night, keeps his mouth open and has a dull, apathetic expression, his nose and throat should be examined, and if advisable his tonsils and adenoids should be removed.

DEFECTIVE HEARING.--Permanent deafness among children in the great majority of cases comes from trouble in the throat or nose; hence the most effective measure to prevent deafness is to make sure that every child's nose, throat, and mouth are in a normal condition. Sensitive or timid children try to hide infirmities of any kind, but deaf children seem peculiarly unable to explain their difficulties. "No one," says Cornell, "has ever recorded that a small child complained of inability to hear." A child's ears should be examined if he breathes through his mouth, if he stoops habitually, if he is persistently inattentive, or if he is vague or stupid in carrying out directions. A child who appears normal at times and inattentive or stupid at other times should also be examined, since he may be deaf in one ear.

Temporary deafness may come from accumulated wax in the ear. The wax should be removed by a doctor; inexpert attempts are likely to cause serious injury to the ear drum. Intermittent deafness may be caused by enlarged tonsils and adenoids. Children thus affected are not infrequently punished for seeming disobedience. Such children are especially liable to street accidents.

DEFECTIVE TEETH have been considered on page 44.

POSTURE.--In childhood the bones are soft and yield with comparative ease to continued strains; hence they often become deformed by bad positions assumed in sitting, standing, or in using the body in other ways. The postures habitually assumed by a child should be noticed and good postures should be insisted upon. But it is not enough to admonish him. The various causes tending to encourage bad positions should be corrected; among them are insufficient illumination of books and work, defective eyesight or hearing, obstructions in breathing, muscular weakness, and low general vitality. Children should have their chairs and tables suited to their size for their work both at home and in school.

[Illustration: FIG. 28.--INCORRECT SITTING POSTURES. (*From Cornell, "Health and Medical Inspection of School Children." F. A. Davis Co., Philadelphia.*)]

[Illustration: FIG. 29.--INCORRECT SITTING POSTURES. (*From Cornell, "Health and Medical Inspection of School Children." F. A. Davis Co., Philadelphia.*)]

[Illustration: FIG. 30.--INCORRECT SITTING POSTURES. (*From Cornell, "Health and Medical Inspection of School Children." F. A. Davis Co., Philadelphia.*)]

[Illustration: FIG. 31.--INCORRECT AND CORRECT STANDING POSTURES. (*From Cornell, "Health and Medical Inspection of School Children," F. A. Davis Co., Philadelphia.*)]

The adjustable chairs and desks now used in schools are a marked improvement upon the school furniture which has caused so many deformities in the past.

[Illustration: FIG. 32.--ROUND SHOULDERS. (*Goldthwait, from Pyle's "Personal Hygiene."*)]

One of the serious deformities caused by habitual faulty posture is curvature of the spine. A curvature not only injures a child's appearance and thus handicaps him in later life, but it brings strains and pressure upon the organs of the chest and abdomen which may seriously impair his health. As curvatures often pass unnoticed in their early stages, every child should be inspected occasionally when all his clothing has been removed, to see whether the weight is borne evenly on both feet, whether the development of the two sides is uniform, and whether the head and shoulders are properly carried. It should be noticed when the child stands, whether one shoulder is higher than the other, whether one shoulder blade projects more than the other, whether one hip is higher than the other, and whether one hand is lower than the other when the arms are hanging at the sides. The child should walk both toward and away from the observer, who should notice whether the child uses the two sides of his body in the same way, and whether he drags or shuffles his feet or has other abnormalities of gait.

[Illustration: FIG. 33.--LATERAL CURVATURE. (*From Bancroft's "Posture of School Children." The Macmillan Co., New York.*)]

[Illustration: FIG. 34.--"WING SHOULDER BLADES IN FORWARD SHOULDERS. (*From Bancroft's "Posture of School Children." The Macmillan Co., New York.*)]

If abnormalities are found, a physician should be consulted. Often corrective exercises are all that is needed, and no one should put braces of any kind upon a child unless they have been prescribed by a physician. No attempt should be made to correct the common tendency of children to toe in or "walk pigeon-toed." Toeing-in is a natural manner of walking during the formative period and tends to strengthen the arch of the foot, while toeing-out tends to weaken the arch and to cause flat foot or broken arches.

PREDISPOSITION TO NERVOUSNESS.--Heredity plays an important rôle in the predisposition to nervousness, so that children of nervous parents are particularly likely to show nervous instability. It is, however, difficult to say in a given case how much of his nervousness a child inherits and how much he acquires by imitating the irritability, the out-breaks of temper, and the other evidences of imperfect emotional control displayed by his nervously disposed parents. On the other hand, even children of nervous predisposition sometimes overcome their defects to some extent by imitating parents who have acquired self-control.

Children predisposed to nervousness should be watched with special care, but they should not be allowed to realize that they are the objects of unusual solicitude. They need the most favorable surroundings that can be obtained, and their general health should be maintained at the highest possible level. Any condition that lowers vitality tends to increase their troubles; nervousness may be caused among children of good inheritance, and increased among others, by poor nutrition, lack of exercise and play out-of-doors, fatigue, loss of sleep, eyestrain, adenoid growths, and the poisons of infectious diseases.

It is characteristic of many nervous children that they are too easily stimulated; they may be excitable, restless, unnaturally quick in moving, over-sensitive to pain and discomfort, easily fatigued, irritable in temper, and unable to control the emotions. They frequently make involuntary motions like grimacing and winking the eyes. Children of low nervous tone, however, are not necessarily excitable. A nervous child may be muscularly weak, awkward in gait, listless, dull, clumsy, forgetful, and inattentive. Such children often suffer from cold hands and feet and from profuse perspiration.

Much can be done for these unfortunate children by removing the cause of their troubles if possible, by giving them simple and wholesome surroundings, by suiting their occupations to their strength, by eliminating mental strain, particularly during the adolescent period, and by training them to control their minds as well as their bodies.

"In addition to the hardening of the body, the education of the child should include measures which increase the resistance of the child against pain and discomforts of various sorts. Every child, therefore, should undergo a gradual process of 'psychic hardening' and be taught to bear with equanimity the pain and discomfort to which everyone sooner or later cannot help but be exposed. What I have said about clothing, cold baths, walking in all weather and at all temperatures, play and exercise in the open air, has a bearing on this point, for a child who has formed good habits in these various directions will have learned many lessons in the steeling of his mind to bear pain and to ignore small discomforts."--(Barker: "Principles of Mental Hygiene Applied to the Management of Children Predisposed to Nervousness.")

CONVALESCENT PATIENTS

After serious or prolonged illness the vitality is generally low and all bodily processes are likely to be depressed. During convalescence, therefore, the digestion is feeble, the muscles are weak so that fatigue follows slight exertion, and the sluggish condition of the circulation renders the patient especially sensitive to cold. Since the nervous system also becomes depressed and irritable, a convalescent patient is easily excited, easily discouraged, and quickly fatigued by mental effort. He finds the simplest decisions hard to make, and his emotions difficult to control; indeed, many a patient who has borne acute pain with unflinching courage becomes peevish at this stage, weeps easily, and expects more expression of sympathy than is good for him. Some persons naturally make quick recoveries, while others recuperate slowly. A long and tedious convalescence, it should be remembered, is the patient's misfortune rather than his fault.

In restoring a convalescent patient to normal living it is imperative to proceed slowly. Food should be increased gradually both in variety and in amount; but the patient's appetite is not always a safe guide, and it may need to be encouraged or to be restrained. Both mental and physical exertion should begin only under careful supervision, and should increase by slow degrees. The patient should sleep as much as possible, should take long intervals of rest, and should continue no occupation to the point of fatigue. A patient who has been ill in a hospital or who has had at home the exclusive services of a nurse or an attendant, often finds the period following his return or following the nurse's departure an exceedingly difficult transition. The family should not expect or allow him to resume too many duties at a time when the mere acts of bathing and dressing may demand all the strength he has. Many convalescents are obliged, or think they are obliged, to take up regular work again before their strength is fully restored. There is generally no economy in so doing; indeed, time is saved in the end by waiting until recovery is complete before undertaking full work.

Important as it is to build up the patient's physical strength, it is hardly less important to direct his thoughts away from himself and his sickness, and to help him renew his interest in normal living. During his illness he has of necessity relied upon the judgment and support of other persons, and his pain and discomfort have forced him to think constantly of himself and his many needs. The habit of sickness is readily broken by some persons, particularly by those whose nervous exhaustion has not been great and whose interests outside themselves are naturally keen. But the sick point of view has remarkable tenacity, and other patients, unless circumstances or deliberate efforts redirect their thoughts, will look upon themselves as invalids to the end of time.

Hopefulness promotes health, while discouragement, apprehension, and unhappiness lower the tone of the whole system. Hence set backs, failures, delays, and relapses should not be dwelt upon, but signs of progress should be mentioned; judiciously however, since overdone attempts to cheer a patient seldom fail to have the opposite effect. If objects or situations that suggest undesirable thoughts are eliminated, the less often those thoughts tend to recur. Therefore, in order to break the habit of sickness, old thoughts must be gradually banished and new ones must be substituted. Sick-room appliances should be put out of sight as soon as they are no longer needed, and the patient may profit by moving into a different bed room. A few days spent away from home as soon as his strength permits often prove effective in breaking up sickness associations; the patient is generally encouraged when he finds that he can sleep in a different bed, endure some fatigue, and exist without daily visits from the doctor. Even a day spent at a different house in the same town sometimes directs the patient's thoughts into fresh channels. Gradually, but as quickly as safety allows, he should take his place in the normal family life and cease to be treated as an exception.

Merely eliminating associations with sickness, however, is not enough; and exhorting a patient to forget himself and to become interested in something seldom accomplishes anything, especially if he is so depleted by illness that the thought of everyday activities suggests only weariness and pain. A person so weak that he is thoroughly fatigued by dressing himself should not be expected to view with enthusiasm the prospect of a full day's work. Much, however, may be accomplished by providing something that the patient really likes to do, and deliberate efforts must be made to stimulate his interest in some occupation, however simple it may be.

Occupations for invalids are more than a means to pass away the time; they are also of distinct curative value. The patient's interest is not always easy to arouse, and some ingenuity may be needed in the beginning; sometimes interest is best aroused by working at some handicraft in his presence, and finally offering, as a favor, to teach him to do it also. His interest in any occupation is invariably increased if a well person not only directs but shares in the work.

Care should be taken to select occupations suited to the patient's physical condition, to his age, tastes, and mental development. Two or three occupations are better than one, so that he may change from one to another before any one becomes tedious. Work requiring fine motions, close attention, or concentrated thought should be used for short periods, only, and no work should be continued to the point of fatigue. The patient should not be allowed to feel that he must finish a certain amount in a certain time. Even poor work is better than none, and a patient should always be encouraged by judicious praise.

Games and puzzles are useful to some extent, but an aimless occupation is not so beneficial as one which has a tangible product, particularly a product that is useful as well as beautiful. Occupations frequently possible for invalids and convalescents include knitting, crocheting, many kinds of needle work, clay modeling, basketry, stenciling, weaving, book-binding, metal work, and photography. Manuals are now available giving directions for these and many other handicrafts. Sick children often enjoy collecting stamps, post marks, and other objects, making scrap books, sewing, weaving, knitting, paper folding, and various other kindergarten occupations.

CHRONIC PATIENTS

The whole field of caring for the sick offers nowhere greater opportunity for fine and finished work than it offers in the case of chronic invalids. It is an achievement of which an artist might be proud to make a chronic patient comfortable in body, happy in mind, and agreeable to others. Moreover, since success can never be attained by one who wearies in well doing, the care given to a chronic invalid tests not only the attendant's skill but also her moral and spiritual quality.

Care of a chronic patient has for its aims maintaining the patient's health, rendering him as happy and comfortable in mind and body as it is possible for him to be, and providing whatever special treatment and attention his case requires. In order to maintain his health constant attention must be given to diet, to hygiene of the sick room, and indeed to all his surroundings. In many chronic illnesses, such as rheumatism and kidney disease, the diet is prescribed by the doctor; in every case care should be taken that the patient is not overfed or underfed, that the food is suited to his digestive powers, that foods causing flatulence are eliminated, particularly if the patient's trouble is heart disease, and not the least important requirement, that he derive as much pleasure from his food as possible.

The regular daily care of the patient and of his room, already described in this book, should be scrupulously carried out, and no less scrupulously during the tenth year than it was during the tenth day. Cleanliness in every detail is absolutely essential to the patient's welfare; no one is more unpleasant either to himself or to others than a chronic patient who is neglected. Patients who are constantly in bed, it should be remembered, and paralyzed patients in particular, are peculiarly susceptible to pressure sores. If a patient is able, it is extremely important for him to sit up in a chair part of the day. Sitting up should never be omitted because it involves the expenditure of time and trouble for the attendant.

It is often said that for most people some personal experience of sickness is beneficial; it can safely be said, however, that no one benefits from spending any considerable portion of his life in a state of helplessness and suffering. Behavior and character itself are determined by influences constantly coming into the mind from daily surroundings and associations with other people: one who recalls this fact needs only a moment's reflection to realize how ill adapted to healthy development of mind and character are the limited lives of the sick. Especially unfortunate is the situation of chronic invalids, shut off as they are from the objective interests and activities of normal life, deprived of all practice in making the salutary small adjustments and sacrifices required in every day living with other people, and self-centered as they necessarily tend to become from the inevitable focusing of attention upon their own discomforts and pain.

On the whole, a surprisingly large number of invalids successfully resist the disintegrating effects of sickness upon character. But it is nevertheless true, as Dr. Weir Mitchell says, that "Sickness ennobles a few but debases many." A selfish invalid has more than once destroyed the happiness of an entire family, or spoiled the life of one member of it by monopolizing her whole time and attention. Families should remember that their injudicious sacrifices seldom bring enduring happiness or contentment to the patient himself; indeed, in the long run such sacrifices generally injure him even more than they injure his victims. Clearly much must and should be sacrificed by members of a family to the needs of an invalid; but in general it may be said that a sacrifice is injudicious if it relieves the patient of activity or responsibility that he can support without injury, if it makes him more dependent in mind or body, if it results in restricting his attention to himself and his affairs, or if it increases his tendency to make demands on others.

Purposeful activity of some sort and the necessity for contributing to the welfare of others are essential parts of a wholesome life. If these essentials are entirely eliminated from the life of an invalid, the patient's greatest needs are probably left unsatisfied, even though the physical care he receives may be perfect in every detail. All that was said in regard to occupations for invalids applies with particular force to occupations for chronic patients, since however valuable manual occupations may be as a means to bring about recovery, they are still more valuable in furnishing interest and purpose in a life whose only prospect is a succession of weary, useless years. Handicapped patients sometimes learn occupations that yield a financial return, and ability to earn even a little stimulates self respect and mental health, whether the money is needed or not. The important point, however, is that the finished product should have a recognized use.

In addition to enabling the patient to make things with his hands, a way should be found if possible by which he may contribute to the group of people with whom he lives. If a way can be discovered for him to do so, the opportunity should not be denied him nor should his service fail to be noted and appreciated, even if it is nothing more than telling a story to a restless child.

CARE OF THE AGED

At the end of life, as at its beginning, every individual especially needs the interest and protection of his own family. In ordinary circumstances neither a baby nor an aged person can be cared for so fittingly or so successfully in any other place as he can be in his own home.

With advancing years is to be expected a general slowing down of all the powers. In old age both body and mind show characteristic changes, and particularly changes causing lowered resistance and diminished vigor. If the manner of living is adapted to these changes, both happiness and usefulness may be prolonged. But so gradually do the changes often come that they may escape notice for a long time, and the younger generation in looking back sometimes realizes with regret how much earlier measures might have been taken to prolong the usefulness and to mitigate the discomforts of aged parents and friends.

Old people are keenly sensitive to cold, since the circulation gradually becomes less vigorous and they take little exercise. Keeping them warm both in bed and out adds more perhaps to their comfort than any other one measure. They should have warm underclothing and soft shawls and other extra wraps. A real service will be rendered by the person who invents a suitable and dignified wrap for old or feeble men, who dislike the informality of sweaters and feel disgraced by shawls. Old persons should and can be kept warm in bed, by providing them with hot water bags, with warm night clothes including stockings, by using woollen or outing flannel sheets if necessary, and by providing a sufficient number of light but warm bed covers. It is not always understood that many covers do not remedy the deficiencies of a thin mattress. If a thick mattress or two thin mattresses cannot be provided, a thick comforter or even many layers of newspaper should be placed between the mattress and the springs, and another thick comforter should be placed between the mattress and the lower sheet. Rubbing the body with warm olive oil often affords great comfort, by improving the circulation and thus increasing the sensation of warmth, and also by relieving the tendency of the skin to become dry and cracked. Poor circulation at night may cause cramps in the muscles of the legs; the cramps can usually be relieved by warmth and gentle rubbing.

Old people frequently wish their rooms to be very hot, both by day and by night, even as hot as 80° or 85°, but if it is possible to keep them warm in any other way the temperature of the room should be kept at 70°. Well ventilated rooms are highly important for old people as for all others of low resistance, and it is entirely possible for their rooms to be warm and yet well ventilated. Aged persons should be carefully guarded from chill, exposure, crowds, and infected persons. Like little children they are peculiarly susceptible to the respiratory diseases, which cause many of the deaths commonly attributed to old age.

Digestion usually becomes weaker than in earlier years, and less food is needed. It should be simple, hot, and divided into four or five meals rather than three. Old people often wake at an early hour, and hot nourishment will prevent them from growing weak and faint while waiting for the family breakfast. Both constipation and looseness of the bowels are common ailments in old age. So far as possible the bowels should be regulated by means of diet; but muscular weakness resulting in inability to control the bowels should not be mistaken for and treated as diarrhoea.

It is unwise for old people to undertake unaccustomed or sudden muscular exertion, since the muscular system including the heart muscle grows weak and is generally unable to endure great strain. The bones, moreover, grow brittle and heal with difficulty if broken, so that persons of advanced years no matter how active should avoid walking on icy pavements, climbing on chairs to reach high shelves, and placing themselves in other insecure positions. Assistance must be tactfully given, however, as active old people are inclined to resent it. On the other hand, old people should be encouraged to continue moderate and safe activities, and to take regular exercises suited to their strength. Although increasing muscular weakness tends to make most old people indolent, it is far better for them both in mind and in body to remain as active as they can without danger of too great fatigue. At all events, they should be prevented if possible from becoming bedridden.

Since in old age sight, hearing, and other special senses become less acute, one should remember that an old person may not notice the odor of escaping gas, the light of a smouldering match, or the sound of an approaching motor car, and that he must be specially guarded from such dangers of every day life. On account of their dulled perceptions old people are sometimes unjustly considered to be less intelligent than they really are. Young people moreover should be told, if an aged person is untidy and careless in personal habits, that the apparent negligence is caused by dulled perceptions and diminished muscular control for which old people are no more responsible than they are for failing eyesight or for inability to hear.

Families should also realize that changes in mind and character are beyond an aged person's control and that they should not be made the cause for remonstrance or arguing. Just as the arteries harden with advancing years, as the bones become brittle and as other tissues become less flexible, so changes are likely to occur in the nervous system. It is not surprising when the brain substance like other tissues is becoming less flexible, that the powers of attention should weaken, that memory for recent events should diminish, or that other mental powers should fail. Changes in disposition are not uncommon: previously controlled persons sometimes become querulous and exacting, while excitable and irritable persons become more placid. With most old people emotions become less intense; feeble old people hardly realize great joy or great sorrow, and seldom look forward to death with apprehension.

Among the most important changes that occur in the nervous system is its gradual loss in power to respond to new demands. New habits are difficult or impossible to form, and old habits are hard to break. Attempts to break the habits of a life time are therefore dangerous, and radical changes in old people's ways of living are attended by risk as well as by unhappiness. Such loss of adaptability in the nervous system makes it increasingly difficult for old people to assimilate new ideas and to understand new points of view. The feeling that the world is strange and that the next generation has gone on without them accounts for the tragic loneliness of many old people. Clearly it is for those who are younger and more flexible to bridge the gulf between the generations by their understanding and their sympathy.

Physical care to whatever extent it is needed should be given to all old people as soon as they are unable to care for themselves, and thought should be given to adapting their surroundings and ways of living to their strength and needs, just as they should be adapted to the strength and needs of chronic patients. But a warning should be given against managing old people too much. It is hard for people who have managed their own lives successfully for many years to be managed, even for their own good. Indeed, it is questionable kindness to deprive old people of all freedom of action, even if following their own inclinations occasionally has disastrous results. Few persons would wish to prolong their lives if long life involved being thwarted in every desire, and sometimes real kindness consists in allowing old people to do certain things that are not good for them. Keeping them warm and letting them do as they please will go far to make old people happy.

Many of the changes in old age reverse the developing process of childhood. In youth and age extremes meet, and the care of the aged presents certain marked similarities to the care of little children. Both require simple food, occupations suited to their strength, and protection from infections, from fatigue, and from nervous strain; both are dependent, more or less helpless, and for their happiness both need the affectionate care of their own families. But in one respect their needs are fundamentally different. In childhood formation of proper habits is all important, and in caring for children the future effect of every word and act must be taken into consideration. Old people, on the other hand, since they live largely in the past and their habits are irrevocably formed, may be indulged without harm in ways that would demoralize a child; with a clear conscience one may make them happy in ways both great and small. This difference makes possible one of the greatest pleasures that come to one who cares for the helpless and the sick, for of all enduring satisfactions few are greater than the power to fill with comfort and happiness the closing days of life.

EXERCISES

1. What is meant by a physical defect? Name some of the most common defects.

2. Name some permanent injuries to the body caused by defective teeth; by diseased or enlarged tonsils and adenoids; by faulty posture.

3. Describe some common symptoms of eye strain in children; of enlarged tonsils and adenoids; of deafness.

4. Name several possible causes of round shoulders, and explain why urging a round-shouldered child to hold himself erect is seldom enough to make him correct his posture.

5. What measures should be taken to overcome nervousness in children?

6. Describe in detail the health work carried on in the public schools of your city or town. Considering the important part played by uncorrected physical defects in causing permanent physical disability among adults, do you think in the long run it is cheaper or more expensive for a community to spend money in protecting the health of school children?

7. Discuss the particular needs of convalescent and of chronic patients.

8. Explain the effect of activity upon recovery, and explain why it is desirable for invalids to have occupation.

9. What special needs should be provided for in caring for old people?

FOR FURTHER READING

Invalid Occupations--Tracy.

Occupation Therapy--Dunton.

Handicrafts for the Handicapped--Hall and Buck.

When Mother Lets Us Make Toys--Rich.

Amusements for Convalescent Children--New York State Department of Health, Albany.

Essentials of Medicine--Emerson, Chapter IX.

Civics and Health--Allen.

How to Live--Fisher and Fisk, Chapter III, Section II; and Supplementary Notes, Section III.

Health Work in the Schools--Hoag and Terman.

Medical Inspection of Schools--Gulick and Ayres.

The Hygiene of the Child--Terman.

Posture of School Children--Bancroft.

CHAPTER XV

QUESTIONS FOR REVIEW

I. Show how you would:

1. Make an unoccupied bed. (Notice the number of minutes it takes you to do it well.)

2. Remove all the covers from an unoccupied bed and leave the bed to air.

3. Open a bed to receive a patient.

II. Show how you would:

1. Change all the linen and remake an occupied bed. (How long did it take you?)

2. Turn a patient from his back to his side, and the reverse.

3. Remove, shake, and readjust a patient's pillows.

4. Move a patient from one bed to another.

5. Prepare a weak patient to sit up in a chair, and assist him from the bed to the chair.

6. Assist a weak patient from the chair to the bed.

7. Arrange pillows and back rest for a patient to sit up in bed; and also how you would remove the pillows and back rest.

III. Show how you would:

1. Lift a patient who has slipped down toward the foot of the bed, and show what you would do to prevent him from slipping down.

2. Prevent bed covers from resting upon a sensitive foot, leg, abdomen, or arm.

3. Describe and demonstrate every device you would use and every thing you would do to prevent pressure sores.

4. Arrange pillows to support the arms of a person sitting up in bed.

5. Arrange a table or a substitute for a table to support the book or work of a patient sitting up in bed.

6. Arrange the light for a patient who is allowed to read in bed.

IV.

1. Assemble all the articles you would use in giving a bed bath. (How long did it take you?)

2. Show how to give a complete bed bath. (How long did it take you? Did you have to stop the bath to fetch anything you had forgotten?)

3. What special care would you give to the mouth and teeth? to the finger and toe nails? to the hair? to badly tangled hair? How would you cleanse the mouth of a helpless patient?

4. Show how to shampoo the hair of a bed patient.

5. Show how you would give a bath to a baby.

6. Show everything that you would do to prepare a patient for the night.

V.

1. Show how to take the temperature, pulse, and respiration.

2. Show how to cleanse a clinical thermometer.

3. Show how to give a foot bath (*a*) to a patient out of bed, (*b*) to a patient in bed.

4. Show how you would give a cool sponge bath to a feverish patient.

5. Show how to give, remove, and cleanse a bed-pan.

6. Show how to fill and apply a hot water bag; an ice bag.

7. Show how to prepare and apply a mustard paste; a mustard leaf; a flaxseed poultice; hot fomentations; cold compresses.

8. Show how to measure and administer a fluid medicine; pills or tablets.

9. Show how to prepare and administer a salt and water enema to a grown person; to a baby.

10. Show how to prepare steam inhalations.

11. Show how to apply an ointment; a liniment.

VI.

1. Show how you would feed a helpless patient who is lying down.

2. Show how you would feed a patient who is able to sit up but unable to use his hands.

3. Prepare a liquid nourishment tray.

4. Set a tray for light diet; for full diet.

5. Show how to place a tray for a patient unable to sit up but able to feed himself; for a patient sitting up in bed.

6. What personal care should be given a patient just before meals? just after meals?

7. How would you modify the diet of a patient inclined to constipation? to diarrhoea?

VII.

1. Describe effective household methods for removing dust.

2. Demonstrate the cleaning of a refrigerator.

3. Show how to ventilate a sick room while protecting the patient from direct draughts.

4. Show how to clean a sick room with a minimum of disturbance to the patient.

5. Explain how a patient with communicable disease should be isolated.

6. Demonstrate the daily care of a room occupied by a patient with communicable disease.

7. Explain methods of concurrent disinfection.

8. Explain methods of terminal disinfection.

9. Tell how the following should be disinfected: discharges from the nose, throat, eyes, ears, bowels, bladder, wounds, and sores; bed and personal linen; blankets; mattresses; dishes; utensils, especially bedpans and urinals; clothing and person of the attendant, especially the hands; furniture, rugs, and woodwork.

VIII.

1. Name some of the most obvious symptoms of sickness.

2. Name some symptoms that would lead you to take a patient to a doctor; to send for a doctor; to send for a doctor in haste.

3. Name some symptoms that are dangerous to neglect even though the patient feels fairly well.

4. What are some of the symptoms of physical defects in children? Name some conditions that are frequently caused by unremedied defects.

5. Name some diseases commonly ushered in by symptoms resembling those of a cold in the head.

6. What symptoms would lead you to isolate a patient?

7. Give as many illustrations as you can of the part played by good and bad habits in determining health and sickness.

IX.

1. How would you dress a cut? a burn? a sprain?

2. What would you do for a person suffering from colic? nausea? diarrhoea? chill?

3. What are the symptoms of shock? heat stroke? heat prostration? What treatment would you give in each case?

4. What would you do for a fainting person? for a person suffering from nose bleed? from earache? from a cinder in the eye?

5. What course of action would you advise for a person troubled with sleeplessness? frequent headaches? excessive irritability? unusual depression of spirits? unfounded suspicions of other persons' motives? a tendency to have the feelings hurt easily? inability to control the emotions?

X.

1. Why is it better to prevent sickness than to cure it?

2. Name the essentials of good hygienic conditions for babies, for children, for grown people, for the aged.

3. How much of the sickness in the United States is preventable?

4. If part of the sickness is preventable, why is it not prevented?

5. What constitutes adequate care of the sick?

6. What proportion of the young men in your community who were drafted have been rejected for physical disability? How many were rejected for disabilities that might have been prevented?

XI. (Answers to the following questions can generally be obtained from local health officers.)

1. What are the duties and powers of your local board of health?

2. How much did your city or town spend per person last year on health protection? How does this amount compare with the amount spent per person for police protection? for fire protection?

3. Who inspects the water supply in your town? the milk supply? the food supply?

4. In your city, what was the number of deaths per 100,000 of the population from tuberculosis each year for the last five years? from typhoid fever?

5. Is there a tuberculosis sanitarium in your city or county? Are nurses employed to supervise tuberculosis patients who remain at home?

6. What provision does your community make for patients suffering from other communicable diseases?

7. What measures are taken in your community to instruct school children in matters of health? to instruct grown persons?

8. How does your community provide medical and nursing care for persons unable to pay part or all of the cost of such service?

XII. Explain why the following common beliefs are erroneous or unfounded:

1. That a damp cellar causes diphtheria.

2. That night air is harmful.

3. That one should "stuff a cold" and "starve a fever."

4. That almost everyone needs a tonic in the spring.

5. That the health of one's family would be endangered if a tuberculosis hospital were placed on the next block.

6. That clearing up the back yard will protect the children of a family from infantile paralysis.

7. That odorless and tasteless water is necessarily free from harmful germs.

8. That all children should have the children's diseases, and have them as early as possible.

9. That boils are a benefit to the system by removing impurities from the blood.

10. That tomatoes cause cancer.

11. That consumption is inherited.

12. That dirt breeds disease.

13. That diseases come up drains.

14. That if a teaspoonful of medicine does you good, a tablespoonful will do you more good.

15. That instinct teaches a mother how to care for her baby.

16. That low heeled shoes, though suitable for boys and men, cause broken arches in women and girls.

17. That in one's own case, the rule that everyone needs regular meals, regular hours of sleep, and daily exercise out of doors, may be safely violated.

APPENDIX

The New York City Department of Health has kindly permitted us to include the following circulars of information issued by the Division of Child Hygiene.

DEPARTMENT OF HEALTH THE CITY OF NEW YORK

INSTRUCTIONS TO PARENTS REGARDING THE CARE OF THE MOUTH AND TEETH.

The physical examination of school children shows that in many instances the teeth are in a decayed and unhealthy condition.

Decayed teeth cause an unclean mouth. Toothache and disease of the gums may result.

Neglect of the first teeth is a frequent cause of decay of the second teeth.

If a child has decayed teeth, it cannot properly chew its food. Improperly chewed food and an unclean mouth cause bad digestion, and consequently poor general health.

If a child is not in good health, it cannot keep up with its studies in school. It is more likely to contract any contagious disease, and it has not the proper chance to grow into a robust, healthy adult.

If the child's teeth are decayed, it should be taken to a dentist at once.

The teeth should be brushed after each meal, using a tooth brush and tooth powder.

The following tooth powder is recommended:

2 oz. powdered precipitated chalk. ½ oz. powdered Castile soap, 1 dram powdered orris root. Thoroughly mix.

This prescription can be filled by any druggist at a cost not to exceed fifteen cents.

DEPARTMENT OF HEALTH CITY OF NEW YORK

Instructions to Parents Regarding the Care of the Nose

The physical examination of school children shows that in many instances they breathe through the mouth because they cannot breathe properly or sufficiently through the nose.

This may be due to bad habits in regard to keeping the nose clean, or, in a majority of instances, to a growth which is known as "adenoids" and which stops up the back of the nose. In either case, the air is not breathed through the nose, and the child becomes what is known as a "mouth breather."

Constant breathing through the mouth causes the child to become pale, restless in its sleep and dull in its actions. The child often speaks as though it had a cold in the head. Frequently there is an almost constant discharge from the nose.

Mouth breathing renders a child especially liable to contract tuberculosis and other infectious diseases; in fact, the child has very little resistance to disease of any kind.

Every child should be given a handkerchief, and be taught to thoroughly blow the nose several times each day. If, after doing this regularly, the child is still unable to breathe properly through the nose, it is probable that an adenoid growth is present. Such children should be taken to the family physician or to a dispensary for further advice and treatment.

Do not wait too long in the hope that the child will outgrow the condition, for the effect of adenoid growths persisting throughout childhood may injure the person for life.

Have your child's throat and nose examined one month after measles, scarlet fever, or diphtheria.

DEPARTMENT OF HEALTH CITY OF NEW YORK

Instructions to Parents on the Care of Children's Hair and Scalp

Children affected with vermin of the head are excluded from school. The following directions will cure the condition:

Mix one-half pint of sweet oil and one-half pint of kerosene oil. Shake the mixture well and saturate the hair with the mixture. Then wrap the head in a large bath towel or rubber cap so that the head is entirely covered; the head must remain covered from six to eight hours.

(Tincture of larkspur may be used instead of oil mixture. The directions for use are the same.)

After removing the towel, the head should be shampooed as follows:

To two quarts of warm water add one teaspoonful of sodium carbonate (washing soda). Wet the hair with this solution and then apply Castile soap and rub the head thoroughly about ten minutes. Wash the soap out of the hair with repeated washings of clear warm water. Dry the hair thoroughly.

Nits: If the head is shampooed regularly each week as above described, it will cure and prevent the condition of "nits."

DEPARTMENT OF HEALTH CITY OF NEW YORK

DIET FOR CHILD FROM 12TH TO 18TH MONTH

FIRST MEAL--ON RISING.

(1) 1 to 2 ounces juice of a sweet orange

or

Pulp of 6 stewed prunes

or

1 ounce pineapple juice.

(2) 8 ounces milk with either zwieback, or toasted biscuits or stale toasted bread.

Note: Fruit must be given either ½ hour before or ½ hour after milk.

SECOND MEAL--DURING FORENOON.

Milk alone or with zwieback.

NOON MEAL.

(1) 6 ounces soup

or

3 ounces beef juice.

Note: Soup may be made of chicken, beef or mutton.

(2) Stale bread may be added to the above.

FOURTH MEAL--AFTERNOON.

Milk or toasted bread and milk.

EVENING MEAL.

(1) 4 ounces thick gruel mixed with 4 ounces top half milk.

Taken with zwieback.

Note: Gruel may be made of oatmeal, farina, barley, hominy, wheatena, or rice.

(2) Apple sauce

or

Prune jelly.

Total milk in 24 hours, 1 to 1¼ quarts.

Note: 8 ounces is equal to a half pint.

DEPARTMENT OF HEALTH CITY OF NEW YORK

DIET FOR CHILD FROM 18TH TO 24TH MONTH

BREAKFAST.

(1) Juice of one sweet orange

or

Pulp of six stewed prunes

or

Pineapple juice (fresh or bottled) 1 ounce.

(2) A cereal such as cream of wheat, oatmeal, farina, or hominy preparations with top milk (top 16 ounces) sweetened or salted. A glass of milk, bread and butter.

Note: If constipated give the fruit ½ hour before breakfast with water; if not, they may be given during the forenoon.

Raw fruit juice must be given either ½ hour before or ½ hour after milk.

FORENOON.

A glass of milk with two toasted biscuits or zwieback or graham crackers.

DINNER.

(1) Broth or soup made of beef, mutton, or chicken, and thickened with peas, farina, sago or rice

or

Beef juice with stale bread crumbs; or clear vegetable soup with yolk of egg

or

Egg soft boiled, with bread crumbs, or the egg poached, with a glass of milk.

(2) Dessert: apple sauce, prune pulp, with stale lady-fingers or graham wafers

or

Plain puddings: rice, bread, tapioca, blanc-mange, junket or baked custard.

SUPPER.

Glass of milk, warm or cold; zwieback and custard or stewed fruit.

Total milk in 24 hours, 1½ quarts.

DEPARTMENT OF HEALTH

CITY OF NEW YORK

DIET FOR CHILD FROM TWO TO THREE YEARS

BREAKFAST.

(1) Juice of 1 sweet orange

or

Pulp of 6 stewed prunes

or

1 ounce pineapple juice (fresh or bottled)

or

Apple sauce.

(2) A cereal such as oatmeal, farina, cream of wheat, hominy or rice, slightly sweetened or salted as preferred, with the addition of top milk (top 16 ounces)

or

A soft boiled or poached egg with stale bread or toast.

(3) A glass of milk.

Note: If constipated give the fruit ½ hour before breakfast with water; if not, they may be given during the forenoon.

Milk and raw fruit juice must not be given at same meal.

DINNER.

(1) Broth or soup made of chicken, mutton or beef, thickened with arrowroot, split peas, rice, or with addition of the yolk of an egg or toast squares.

(2) Scraped beef or white meat of chicken, or broiled fish (small amount)

or

Mashed or baked potatoes with fresh peas or spinach or carrots.

(3) Dessert: apple sauce, baked apple, rice pudding, junket or custard.

SUPPER.

(1) A cereal or egg (if egg is not taken with breakfast) with stale bread or toast

or

Bread and milk or bread and cocoa or bread and custard.

(2) Stewed fruit.

DEPARTMENT OF HEALTH

CITY OF NEW YORK

DIET FOR CHILD FROM THREE TO SIX YEARS

BREAKFAST.

(1) Fruits: an orange, apple, pear or stewed prunes.

(2) Cereal: oatmeal, hominy, rice or wheat preparations, well cooked and salted, with thin cream and sugar

or

Egg: soft boiled, poached, omelet or scrambled.

(3) Milk or cocoa.

DINNER.

(1) Soup: beef, chicken or mutton.

(2) Meat: chicken or beefsteak or roast beef or lamb chops or fish.

(3) Vegetables: spinach or carrots or string beans, peas, cauliflower tops, mashed or baked potatoes, beets or lettuce (without vinegar)

Macaroni, spaghetti.

Bread and butter--not fresh bread or rolls.

(4) Dessert: custard, rice or bread or tapioca pudding, ice cream (once a week) cornstarch pudding (chocolate or other flavor) stewed prunes or baked apple.

SUPPER.

(1) Milk toast or graham crackers and milk

or

A thick soup, as pea, or cream of celery with bread and butter

or

A cereal and thin cream with bread and butter.

(2) Stewed fruit; custard or plain pudding; jam or jelly.

GLOSSARY

(For complete definitions of the following words the student is referred to general and scientific dictionaries)

A

ANTISEPTIC.--A substance which prevents or hinders the growth of micro-organisms.

ANTITOXIN.--A substance that neutralizes the action of a toxin.

ASEPTIC.--Free from living germs.

AXILLA.--The armpit.

B

BACILLUS (pl. bacilli).--A rod-shaped or elongated bacterium.

BACTERIAL.--Relating to bacteria.

BACTERICIDE.--An agent having the power to destroy bacteria.

BACTERIOLOGICAL.--Relating to bacteriology.

BACTERIOLOGY.--The science dealing with microorganisms.

BACTERIUM (pl. bacteria).--A unicellular vegetable micro-organism.

C

CARRIER.--An apparently healthy person who harbors pathogenic germs in his body.

COCCUS (pl. cocci).--A bacterium of spherical or nearly spherical shape.

COUNTER-IRRITANT.--A substance or agent which if applied to the skin causes irritation and thereby relieves an abnormal condition in another part of the body.

D

DEGENERATION.--A deterioration in cells or tissues of the body so that they become less able to perform their proper functions.

DEGENERATIVE.--Pertaining to degeneration.

DEODORANT.--An agent that destroys odors.

DIGESTIVE TRACT.--The entire alimentary canal, including the mouth, oesophagus, stomach, and the small and large intestines.

DIPLOCOCCUS.--A form of coccus in which two individuals remain attached after cell division has taken place.

DISINFECT.--To destroy the germs of disease.

DISINFECTANT.--An agent that destroys the germs of disease.

DISINFECTION.--The process of destroying the germs of disease.

E

EMETIC.--A substance used to induce vomiting.

ENEMA.--An injection of fluid into the rectum.

F

FECAL.--Pertaining to feces.

FECES.--Matter discharged from the bowels; bowel movement.

FERMENTATION.--Decomposition produced in an organic substance by the action of certain living agents.

FISSION.--The process by which a cell divides into two parts.

FLAGELLUM (pl. flagella).--A long hair-like appendage, by the action of which certain micro-organisms are enabled to move.

FLEX.--To bend at a joint.

FOMENTATION.--See *Stupe*.

G

GASTRIC JUICE.--The fluid secreted by the glands of the stomach.

GERM.--A minute unicellular organism, either animal or vegetable; a micro-organism; a microbe.

GERMICIDE.--An agent having the power to kill germs.

H

HOST.--An animal or plant in or upon which another organism lives.

I

IMMUNE.--Not susceptible to a particular disease; also, a person who is not susceptible to a particular disease.

IMMUNITY.--The state in which an individual is not susceptible to a particular disease.

IMMUNIZE.--To render immune.

INCUBATION.--The interval between exposure to an infectious disease and the first appearance of symptoms.

INFECT.--To communicate disease germs.

INFECTION.--An agent by which disease may be communicated from one individual to another; also, an infectious disease.

INOCULATE.--To introduce any biological product directly into the tissues of the body.

INOCULATION.--The process of inoculating.

INTESTINAL TRACT.--The small and large intestines.

M

MICROBE.--See *Germ.*

MICRO-ORGANISM.--See *Germ.*

MUCUS.--The substance secreted by mucous membranes.

MUCOUS MEMBRANES.--The membranes lining certain cavities of the body, especially the digestive and respiratory tracts.

N

NUTRIENT.--One of several chemical groups to which the essential constituents of food belong.

O

ORGANIC.--Derived from or relating to an organism.

ORGANISM.--An individual that is or has been alive.

P

PARASITE.--An individual that lives in or upon another individual.

PASTEURIZATION.--The process of pasteurizing.

PASTEURIZE.--To subject milk to a temperature of 142°-145° Fahrenheit for thirty minutes.

PATHOGENIC.--Disease-producing.

PERTUSSIS.--Whooping-cough.

PROTEID.--One of the complex nitrogenous substances constituting the essential parts of animal and vegetable tissues.

PROTOZOÖN (pl. protozoa).--An animal organism composed of a single cell.

PUS.--The fluid product of inflammation; matter.

PUTREFACTION.--Decomposition of nitrogenous organic matter brought about by micro-organisms and accompanied by a foul odor.

R

RESISTANCE.--See *Immunity.*

RESPIRATORY TRACT.--The air passages, including the nose, mouth, larynx, trachea, bronchial tubes, and lungs.

S

SAPROPHYTE.--A vegetable organism that lives on decaying organic matter.

SARCINA.--Literally, a bundle. Applied to bacteria grouped in bundles or packets.

SEPTIC.--Putrefying or decomposing; infected by pus-producing bacteria.

SEQUELA.--A disease or unhealthy condition following another disease or unhealthy condition.

SERUM.--The fluid which separates from the clot after blood has coagulated; especially, that containing an antitoxin.

SEWAGE.--Any substance containing urine or fecal matter; also, the substance which passes through sewers.

SPIRILLUM (pl. spirilla).--A variety of bacteria having spirally twisted cells.

SPORE.--A resting stage, characterized by great resistance, into which certain germs enter when conditions become unfavorable for their growth.

SPUTUM.--Spit; expectoration.

STAPHYLOCOCCUS.--A variety of bacteria that group themselves in masses resembling bunches of grapes.

STERILE.--Free from living germs; aseptic.

STERILIZATION.--The process of rendering sterile.

STERILIZE.--To render sterile.

STREPTOCOCCUS.--A variety of bacteria that arrange themselves in chains.

STUPE.--A cloth wrung out of hot water and applied to the surface of the body.

SUSCEPTIBLE.--Lacking resistance to a disease.

SUSCEPTIBILITY.--The condition in which resistance to a disease is low.

T

TETRAD.--A variety of bacteria that arrange themselves in groups of four.

TISSUE.--A collection of cells having the same function.

TOXIN.--A poison produced by the action of micro-organisms.

U

UNICELLULAR.--Composed of a single cell.

UTERUS.--The womb.

V

VACCINATE.--To inoculate with a poison in order to bring about immunity to a disease.

VACCINE.--Any substance which if introduced into the body causes the formation of protective substances.

VOMITUS.--Vomited substances.

INDEX

[Transcriber's Note:

Punctuation errors (e.g. missing period at end of sentence, missing quotation marks, etc.) and letters printed upside down have been corrected without note. Except where noted, inconsistencies in hyphenation, capitalization, and spelling (e.g. travelling and traveling) have not been changed. The original index had numerous errors, such as references to terms that do not appear in the text. Except where noted below, it has been left as printed.

The following corrections were made:

p. viii: Records, 105. to Records, 107. (under Chapter IV)

p. ix: Care of the Patients with Communicable Diseases to Care of Patients with Communicable Diseases (under Chapter XII)

p. ix: Care of liver, 251. to Care of linen, 251. (under Chapter XII)

p. 15: innoculation to inoculation (Vaccination and inoculation have saved thousands of lives.)

p. 16: principle to principal (principal causes which diminish resistance), to match cited text

p. 37: gerns to germs (through which disease germs)

p. 40: From "*The Human Mechanism.*" to *From "The Human Mechanism."* (to match format of other captions)

p. 41: perferably to preferably (preferably, chloride of lime.)

p. 77: runnnig to running (thoroughly cleansed under running water)

p. 82: symptons to symptoms (other symptoms of distress)

p. 96: thay to they (taken together they are)

p. 108: 8:30 to 8:30 a.m.

p. 111: develope to develop (may develop into cancer)

p. 115: missing degree symbol added (At noon his temperature was 101°)

p. 132: illnes to illness (unless his illness is slight)

p. 136: servicable to serviceable (makes a serviceable cover)

p. 150: paitent to patient (ready for the patient.)

p. 150-151: removed duplication of text in captions for Fig. 14 and Fig. 15 (CHANGING THE DRAW SHEET, and CHANGING A PATIENT FROM ONE BED TO ANOTHER)

p. 161: erroneous italics removed from "patient" and "her" (even a patient unable to sit up can brush her teeth)

p. 167: added missing "bath" (to give a cool sponge bath)

p. 175: ahould to should (the protection of the abdomen should)

p. 177: expecially to especially (if it is especially difficult or undesirable)

p. 177: patients' to patient's (between the patient's back and the pan;)

p. 178: deoderant to deodorant (a properly kept pan needs no deodorant)

p. 183: invarably to invariably (casual visitors almost invariably offend)

p. 189: nurtients to nutrients (pancreatic juice acts upon all three nutrients)

p. 195: solied to soiled (is always superior to soiled linen.)

p. 205: appy to apply (apply even more strongly to using patent medicines.)

p. 211: 166 to 176 (the directions on page 176.)

p. 216: selzer to seltzer (seltzer aperient)

p. 226: slighest to slightest (there is the slightest possibility of scalding)

p. 227: accidently to accidentally (see that the switch is not accidentally)

p. 228: cohers to coheres (when the mixture coheres)

p. 229: annoint to anoint (anoint it with vaseline)

p. 233: dicharge to discharge (If there is discharge from the eye,)

p. 242: chould to should (visitors should be rigidly)

p. 245: himelf to himself (safeguard the patient himself.)

Table between pp. 246-247: diappearance to disappearance (Two weeks after onset and one week after disappearance)

Table between pp. 246-247: pa-patient to patient (after child last saw patient.)

p. 250: If to It (It may be necessary to provide two bedpans)

p. 266: 216 to 193 (discussed on pages 193 and 52.)

p. 280: etter to better (no better place)

p. 300: attenom, to attention (constant attention must be given)

p. 300: rotion to room, (hygiene of the sick room,)

p. 301: salutory to salutary (making the salutary small adjustments)

p. 308: querelous to querulous (sometimes become querulous)

p. 329: Putrifying to Putrefying (Putrefying or decomposing)

p. 331: bed-cradles to bed cradles (Index sub-entry, under "Appliances")

p. 331: Bed-cradles to Bed cradles (Index entry)

p. 331: Bed-sores to Bed sores (Index entry)

p. 331: Brushburn to Brush burn (Index entry)

p. 332: Foot-bath to Foot bath (Index entry)

p. 333: Microörganisms to Microorganisms (Index entry)

p. 333: Pre-natal to Prenatal (Index entry)

p. 334: oss to loss (Index entry for "Weight, loss of")

A fold-out table was facing p. 247 in the original book. For the plain text versions, it has been split into several smaller tables, with the "DISEASE" column repeated in each section. In the third section, "POLIOMYELITIS" has been hyphenated (POLIO-MYELITIS) to save space.

The footnote pertaining to the table is immediately after it, not at the end of the chapter as usual.

For the Lat-1 and ASCII versions, the oz. symbol has been replaced with oz., and oe ligatures have been changed to oe/OE.]

***** This file should be named 32250-8.txt or 32250-8.zip ***** This
and all associated files of various formats will be found in:
http://www.gutenberg.org/3/2/2/5/32250/

Produced by Heiko Evermann, Fox in the Stars, S.D., and the Online
Distributed Proofreading Team at http://www.pgdp.net

Updated editions will replace the previous one--the old editions will be
renamed.

Creating the works from public domain print editions means that no
one owns a United States copyright in these works, so the Foundation
(and you!) can copy and distribute it in the United States without
permission and without paying copyright royalties. Special rules, set
forth in the General Terms of Use part of this license, apply to copying
and distributing Project Gutenberg-tm electronic works to protect the
PROJECT GUTENBERG-tm concept and trademark. Project
Gutenberg is a registered trademark, and may not be used if you
charge for the eBooks, unless you receive specific permission. If you
do not charge anything for copies of this eBook, complying with the
rules is very easy. You may use this eBook for nearly any purpose
such as creation of derivative works, reports, performances and
research. They may be modified and printed and given away--you may
do practically ANYTHING with public domain eBooks. Redistribution is
subject to the trademark license, especially commercial redistribution.

*** START: FULL LICENSE ***

THE FULL PROJECT GUTENBERG LICENSE PLEASE READ THIS
BEFORE YOU DISTRIBUTE OR USE THIS WORK

To protect the Project Gutenberg-tm mission of promoting the free
distribution of electronic works, by using or distributing this work (or
any other work associated in any way with the phrase "Project
Gutenberg"), you agree to comply with all the terms of the Full Project
Gutenberg-tm License (available with this file or online at
http://gutenberg.net/license).

Section 1. General Terms of Use and Redistributing Project
Gutenberg-tm electronic works

1.A. By reading or using any part of this Project Gutenberg-tm
electronic work, you indicate that you have read, understand, agree to
and accept all the terms of this license and intellectual property
(trademark/copyright) agreement. If you do not agree to abide by all
the terms of this agreement, you must cease using and return or
destroy all copies of Project Gutenberg-tm electronic works in your
possession. If you paid a fee for obtaining a copy of or access to a
Project Gutenberg-tm electronic work and you do not agree to be
bound by the terms of this agreement, you may obtain a refund from
the person or entity to whom you paid the fee as set forth in paragraph
1.E.8.

1.B. "Project Gutenberg" is a registered trademark. It may only be used
on or associated in any way with an electronic work by people who
agree to be bound by the terms of this agreement. There are a few
things that you can do with most Project Gutenberg-tm electronic
works even without complying with the full terms of this agreement.
See paragraph 1.C below. There are a lot of things you can do with
Project Gutenberg-tm electronic works if you follow the terms of this
agreement and help preserve free future access to Project
Gutenberg-tm electronic works. See paragraph 1.E below.

1.C. The Project Gutenberg Literary Archive Foundation ("the
Foundation" or PGLAF), owns a compilation copyright in the collection
of Project Gutenberg-tm electronic works. Nearly all the individual
works in the collection are in the public domain in the United States. If
an individual work is in the public domain in the United States and you
are located in the United States, we do not claim a right to prevent you
from copying, distributing, performing, displaying or creating derivative
works based on the work as long as all references to Project
Gutenberg are removed. Of course, we hope that you will support the
Project Gutenberg-tm mission of promoting free access to electronic
works by freely sharing Project Gutenberg-tm works in compliance with
the terms of this agreement for keeping the Project Gutenberg-tm
name associated with the work. You can easily comply with the terms
of this agreement by keeping this work in the same format with its

attached full Project Gutenberg-tm License when you share it without charge with others.

1.D. The copyright laws of the place where you are located also govern what you can do with this work. Copyright laws in most countries are in a constant state of change. If you are outside the United States, check the laws of your country in addition to the terms of this agreement before downloading, copying, displaying, performing, distributing or creating derivative works based on this work or any other Project Gutenberg-tm work. The Foundation makes no representations concerning the copyright status of any work in any country outside the United States.

1.E. Unless you have removed all references to Project Gutenberg:

1.E.1. The following sentence, with active links to, or other immediate access to, the full Project Gutenberg-tm License must appear prominently whenever any copy of a Project Gutenberg-tm work (any work on which the phrase "Project Gutenberg" appears, or with which the phrase "Project Gutenberg" is associated) is accessed, displayed, performed, viewed, copied or distributed:

This eBook is for the use of anyone anywhere at no cost and with almost no restrictions whatsoever. You may copy it, give it away or re-use it under the terms of the Project Gutenberg License included with this eBook or online at www.gutenberg.net

1.E.2. If an individual Project Gutenberg-tm electronic work is derived from the public domain (does not contain a notice indicating that it is posted with permission of the copyright holder), the work can be copied and distributed to anyone in the United States without paying any fees or charges. If you are redistributing or providing access to a work with the phrase "Project Gutenberg" associated with or appearing on the work, you must comply either with the requirements of paragraphs 1.E.1 through 1.E.7 or obtain permission for the use of the work and the Project Gutenberg-tm trademark as set forth in paragraphs 1.E.8 or 1.E.9.

1.E.3. If an individual Project Gutenberg-tm electronic work is posted with the permission of the copyright holder, your use and distribution must comply with both paragraphs 1.E.1 through 1.E.7 and any additional terms imposed by the copyright holder. Additional terms will be linked to the Project Gutenberg-tm License for all works posted with the permission of the copyright holder found at the beginning of this work.

1.E.4. Do not unlink or detach or remove the full Project Gutenberg-tm License terms from this work, or any files containing a part of this work or any other work associated with Project Gutenberg-tm.

1.E.5. Do not copy, display, perform, distribute or redistribute this electronic work, or any part of this electronic work, without prominently displaying the sentence set forth in paragraph 1.E.1 with active links or immediate access to the full terms of the Project Gutenberg-tm License.

1.E.6. You may convert to and distribute this work in any binary, compressed, marked up, nonproprietary or proprietary form, including any word processing or hypertext form. However, if you provide access to or distribute copies of a Project Gutenberg-tm work in a format other than "Plain Vanilla ASCII" or other format used in the official version posted on the official Project Gutenberg-tm web site (www.gutenberg.net), you must, at no additional cost, fee or expense to the user, provide a copy, a means of exporting a copy, or a means of obtaining a copy upon request, of the work in its original "Plain Vanilla ASCII" or other form. Any alternate format must include the full Project Gutenberg-tm License as specified in paragraph 1.E.1.

1.E.7. Do not charge a fee for access to, viewing, displaying, performing, copying or distributing any Project Gutenberg-tm works unless you comply with paragraph 1.E.8 or 1.E.9.

1.E.8. You may charge a reasonable fee for copies of or providing access to or distributing Project Gutenberg-tm electronic works provided that

- You pay a royalty fee of 20% of the gross profits you derive from the use of Project Gutenberg-tm works calculated using the method you already use to calculate your applicable taxes. The fee is owed to the owner of the Project Gutenberg-tm trademark, but he has agreed to donate royalties under this paragraph to the Project Gutenberg Literary Archive Foundation. Royalty payments must be paid within 60 days following each date on which you prepare (or are legally required to prepare) your periodic tax returns. Royalty payments should be clearly marked as such and sent to the Project Gutenberg Literary Archive Foundation at the address specified in Section 4, "Information about donations to the Project Gutenberg Literary Archive Foundation."

- You provide a full refund of any money paid by a user who notifies you in writing (or by e-mail) within 30 days of receipt that s/he does not agree to the terms of the full Project Gutenberg-tm License. You must require such a user to return or destroy all copies of the works possessed in a physical medium and discontinue all use of and all access to other copies of Project Gutenberg-tm works.

- You provide, in accordance with paragraph 1.F.3, a full refund of any money paid for a work or a replacement copy, if a defect in the electronic work is discovered and reported to you within 90 days of receipt of the work.

- You comply with all other terms of this agreement for free distribution of Project Gutenberg-tm works.

1.E.9. If you wish to charge a fee or distribute a Project Gutenberg-tm electronic work or group of works on different terms than are set forth in this agreement, you must obtain permission in writing from both the Project Gutenberg Literary Archive Foundation and Michael Hart, the owner of the Project Gutenberg-tm trademark. Contact the Foundation as set forth in Section 3 below.

1.F.

1.F.1. Project Gutenberg volunteers and employees expend considerable effort to identify, do copyright research on, transcribe and proofread public domain works in creating the Project Gutenberg-tm collection. Despite these efforts, Project Gutenberg-tm electronic works, and the medium on which they may be stored, may contain "Defects," such as, but not limited to, incomplete, inaccurate or corrupt data, transcription errors, a copyright or other intellectual property infringement, a defective or damaged disk or other medium, a computer virus, or computer codes that damage or cannot be read by your equipment.

1.F.2. LIMITED WARRANTY, DISCLAIMER OF DAMAGES - Except for the "Right of Replacement or Refund" described in paragraph 1.F.3, the Project Gutenberg Literary Archive Foundation, the owner of the Project Gutenberg-tm trademark, and any other party distributing a Project Gutenberg-tm electronic work under this agreement, disclaim all liability to you for damages, costs and expenses, including legal fees. YOU AGREE THAT YOU HAVE NO REMEDIES FOR NEGLIGENCE, STRICT LIABILITY, BREACH OF WARRANTY OR BREACH OF CONTRACT EXCEPT THOSE PROVIDED IN PARAGRAPH F3. YOU AGREE THAT THE FOUNDATION, THE TRADEMARK OWNER, AND ANY DISTRIBUTOR UNDER THIS AGREEMENT WILL NOT BE LIABLE TO YOU FOR ACTUAL, DIRECT, INDIRECT, CONSEQUENTIAL, PUNITIVE OR INCIDENTAL DAMAGES EVEN IF YOU GIVE NOTICE OF THE POSSIBILITY OF SUCH DAMAGE.

1.F.3. LIMITED RIGHT OF REPLACEMENT OR REFUND - If you discover a defect in this electronic work within 90 days of receiving it, you can receive a refund of the money (if any) you paid for it by sending a written explanation to the person you received the work from. If you received the work on a physical medium, you must return the medium with your written explanation. The person or entity that provided you with the defective work may elect to provide a replacement copy in lieu of a refund. If you received the work electronically, the person or entity providing it to you may choose to give you a second opportunity to receive the work electronically in lieu of a refund. If the second copy is also defective, you may demand a refund in writing without further opportunities to fix the problem.

1.F.4. Except for the limited right of replacement or refund set forth in paragraph 1.F.3, this work is provided to you 'AS-IS' WITH NO OTHER

WARRANTIES OF ANY KIND, EXPRESS OR IMPLIED, INCLUDING BUT NOT LIMITED TO WARRANTIES OF MERCHANTIBILITY OR FITNESS FOR ANY PURPOSE.

1.F.5. Some states do not allow disclaimers of certain implied warranties or the exclusion or limitation of certain types of damages. If any disclaimer or limitation set forth in this agreement violates the law of the state applicable to this agreement, the agreement shall be interpreted to make the maximum disclaimer or limitation permitted by the applicable state law. The invalidity or unenforceability of any provision of this agreement shall not void the remaining provisions.

1.F.6. **INDEMNITY**

- You agree to indemnify and hold the Foundation, the trademark owner, any agent or employee of the Foundation, anyone providing copies of Project Gutenberg-tm electronic works in accordance with this agreement, and any volunteers associated with the production, promotion and distribution of Project Gutenberg-tm electronic works, harmless from all liability, costs and expenses, including legal fees, that arise directly or indirectly from any of the following which you do or cause to occur: (a) distribution of this or any Project Gutenberg-tm work, (b) alteration, modification, or additions or deletions to any Project Gutenberg-tm work, and (c) any Defect you cause.

Section 2. Information about the Mission of Project Gutenberg-tm

Project Gutenberg-tm is synonymous with the free distribution of electronic works in formats readable by the widest variety of computers including obsolete, old, middle-aged and new computers. It exists because of the efforts of hundreds of volunteers and donations from people in all walks of life.

Volunteers and financial support to provide volunteers with the assistance they need are critical to reaching Project Gutenberg-tm's goals and ensuring that the Project Gutenberg-tm collection will remain freely available for generations to come. In 2001, the Project Gutenberg Literary Archive Foundation was created to provide a secure and permanent future for Project Gutenberg-tm and future generations. To learn more about the Project Gutenberg Literary Archive Foundation and how your efforts and donations can help, see Sections 3 and 4 and the Foundation web page at http://www.pglaf.org.

Section 3. Information about the Project Gutenberg Literary Archive Foundation

The Project Gutenberg Literary Archive Foundation is a non profit 501(c)(3) educational corporation organized under the laws of the state of Mississippi and granted tax exempt status by the Internal Revenue Service. The Foundation's EIN or federal tax identification number is 64-6221541. Its 501(c)(3) letter is posted at http://pglaf.org/fundraising. Contributions to the Project Gutenberg Literary Archive Foundation are tax deductible to the full extent permitted by U.S. federal laws and your state's laws.

The Foundation's principal office is located at 4557 Melan Dr. S. Fairbanks, AK, 99712., but its volunteers and employees are scattered throughout numerous locations. Its business office is located at 809 North 1500 West, Salt Lake City, UT 84116, (801) 596-1887, email business@pglaf.org. Email contact links and up to date contact information can be found at the Foundation's web site and official page at http://pglaf.org

For additional contact information: Dr. Gregory B. Newby Chief Executive and Director gbnewby@pglaf.org

Section 4. Information about Donations to the Project Gutenberg Literary Archive Foundation

Project Gutenberg-tm depends upon and cannot survive without wide spread public support and donations to carry out its mission of increasing the number of public domain and licensed works that can be freely distributed in machine readable form accessible by the widest array of equipment including outdated equipment. Many small donations ($1 to $5,000) are particularly important to maintaining tax exempt status with the IRS.

The Foundation is committed to complying with the laws regulating charities and charitable donations in all 50 states of the United States. Compliance requirements are not uniform and it takes a considerable effort, much paperwork and many fees to meet and keep up with these requirements. We do not solicit donations in locations where we have not received written confirmation of compliance. To SEND DONATIONS or determine the status of compliance for any particular state visit http://pglaf.org

While we cannot and do not solicit contributions from states where we have not met the solicitation requirements, we know of no prohibition against accepting unsolicited donations from donors in such states who approach us with offers to donate.

International donations are gratefully accepted, but we cannot make any statements concerning tax treatment of donations received from outside the United States. U.S. laws alone swamp our small staff.

Please check the Project Gutenberg Web pages for current donation methods and addresses. Donations are accepted in a number of other ways including including checks, online payments and credit card donations. To donate, please visit: http://pglaf.org/donate

Section 5. General Information About Project Gutenberg-tm electronic works.

Professor Michael S. Hart is the originator of the Project Gutenberg-tm concept of a library of electronic works that could be freely shared with anyone. For thirty years, he produced and distributed Project Gutenberg-tm eBooks with only a loose network of volunteer support.

Project Gutenberg-tm eBooks are often created from several printed editions, all of which are confirmed as Public Domain in the U.S. unless a copyright notice is included. Thus, we do not necessarily keep eBooks in compliance with any particular paper edition.

Most people start at our Web site which has the main PG search facility:

http://www.gutenberg.net

This Web site includes information about Project Gutenberg-tm, including how to make donations to the Project Gutenberg Literary Archive Foundation, how to help produce our new eBooks, and how to subscribe to our email newsletter to hear about new eBooks.

American Red Cross Text-Book on Home
by Jane A. Delano and Anne Hervey Strong and American Red Cross

A free ebook from http://manybooks.net/